MANIC PANIC

LIVING IN COLOR

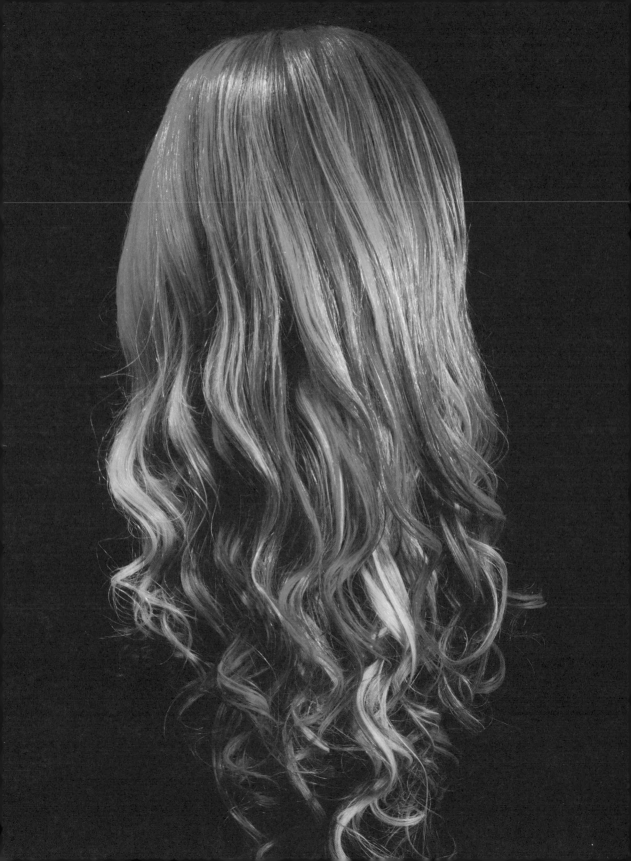

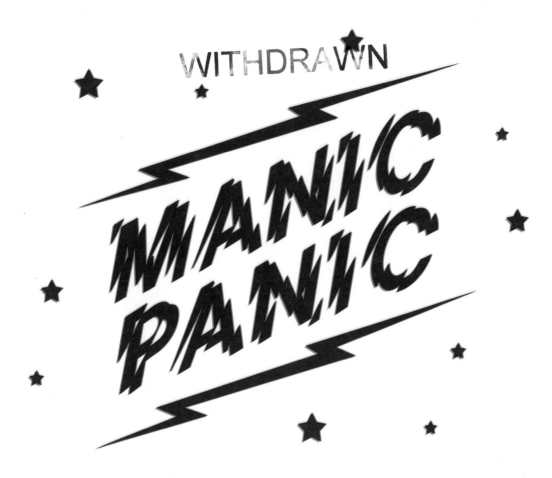

MANIC PANIC

LIVING IN COLOR

A REBELLIOUS GUIDE TO HAIR COLOR AND LIFE

TISH & SNOOKY BELLOMO

WITH JADE TAYLOR

FOREWORD BY RUPAUL

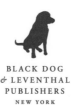

BLACK DOG
& LEVENTHAL
PUBLISHERS
NEW YORK

Black Dog & Leventhal Publishers
Hachette Book Group
1290 Avenue of the Americas
New York, NY 10104
www.hachettebookgroup.com
www.blackdogandleventhal.com

First Edition: October 2019

Black Dog & Leventhal Publishers is an imprint of Perseus
Books, LLC, a subsidiary of Hachette Book Group. The Black
Dog & Leventhal Publishers name and logo are trademarks of
Hachette Book Group, Inc.

The publisher is not responsible for websites (or their
content) that are not owned by the publisher.

The Hachette Speakers Bureau provides a wide range of
authors for speaking events. To find out more, go to
www.HachetteSpeakersBureau.com or call (866) 376-6591.

Print book interior design by Headcase Design.

Library of Congress Cataloging-in-Publication Data has
been applied for.

ISBNs: 978-0-7624-9468-2 (trade paperback);
978-0-7624-9498-9 (ebook)

Printed in China

1010

10 9 8 7 6 5 4 3 2 1

Dedicated to our mother and guardian angel,
Estelle Bellomo

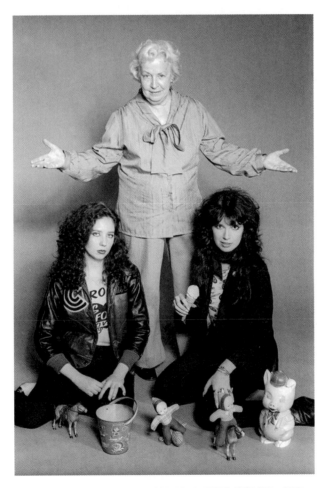

SNOOKY, TISH WITH MOTHER ESTELLE McINNES BELLOMO, 1980
PHOTOGRAPH © MARCIA RESNICK 1980

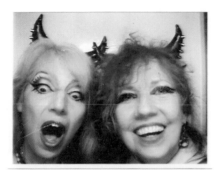
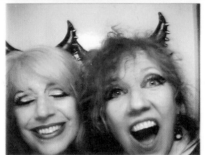
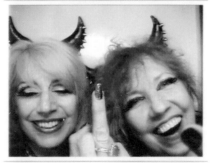
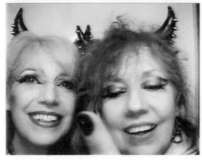

CONTENTS

FOREWORD

Decades ago, before drag was just about anywhere, there were really only a few places that us New York City queens could get what we needed, and one of those places was the Manic Panic store on St. Marks Place, founded by two infamous punk rock singers and scene-stealers, Tish and Snooky Bellomo, formerly of Blondie.

I was first introduced to Tish and Snooky by our mutual friends Randy Barbato and Fenton Bailey around the time we were collaborating on the soundtrack album to my film *Star Booty*. The sisters sang back-up on the album and a thirty-three-year friendship was formed. They backed me up for a performance at The Saint, and we even appeared in a B-52's music video together.

I'll never forget us all waiting on the corner for the production bus to take us to the location while traffic stood at a standstill. People gawked as I towered over the sidewalk during rush hour at Fifty-Second Street and Third Avenue in full drag. I didn't get quite the reception then that I would today.

What I've always admired about Tish and Snooky is their commitment to honoring self-expression. It's a commitment I share. You can be sure we'll all continue to infuse the world with color and glamour for generations to come.

—RuPaul

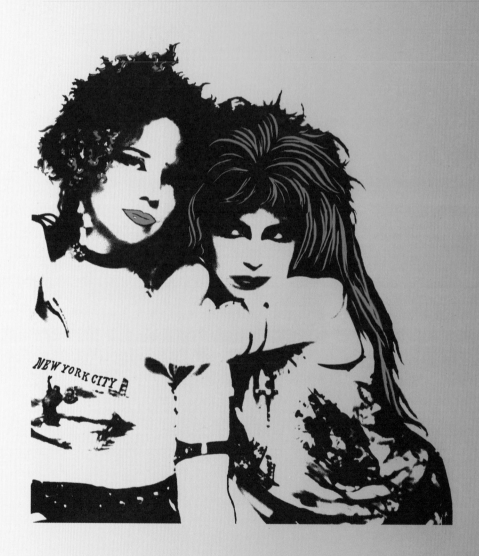

WE DON'T JUST SELL IT, WE LIVE IT

f you had told us back in 1977 that doing what we loved and sharing our unique style would influence music, art, fashion, and beauty for the next four decades, we would've thought you were as crazy as us!

Before Manic Panic was ever a punk rock dream, we were two young, free-spirited NYC sisters who embraced the underground scene, singing at all the local dives and creating our own fashion looks while hanging out with our ultra-fabulous downtown friends.

We grew up without money. Our single mother taught us how to make the best out of whatever we had, using every resource available. Although we never fit in, we were certainly two of the most unusual-looking poor kids in the Bronx. I (Tish) would repurpose outdated hand-me-downs because I liked to sew and design, and I was embarrassed to wear long skirts when minis were in style. Some of my "creations" came out looking quite interesting, to say the least! And Snooky would wear anything and everything people gave us. Stripes? Polka dots mixed with unmatched plaids? No problem!

We remember once seeing our mother perched on the kitchen counter, hanging up some old curtains using a string because we couldn't afford a curtain rod. She turned to us and said, "Don't ever be poor." At that time, we actually

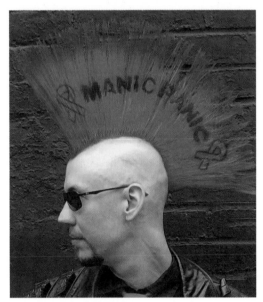

PHOTO BY RENAN BARROSO FOR MANIC PANIC

MANIC PANIC'S OWN MOHAWK DAVE'S ICONIC ROCK 'N' ROLL RED MOHAWK, EMBLAZONED WITH OUR LOGO USING ROCKABILLY BLUE AMPLIFIED COLOR SPRAY

thought that our neighbors who were on welfare were rich! Being poor didn't matter; we thought it was amazing that our mother had invented a rod-less way to hang curtains! Our mother's creativity and resourcefulness inspired us throughout our lives and especially when we opened Manic Panic, the first punk boutique in the United States!

WASTE NOT, WANT NOT

To this day, we never waste anything. Even if a run of hair dye ends up being slightly "off spec" (too dark or too light), we don't compromise on color, but we don't throw it away either. We add it to the "attractive failures/Manic Mix-ups" collection; give it a new name, description, and explanation; and offer it at a discount to our fans who love one-of-a-kind colors and appreciate a good deal. While a shade might not be an exact match to a standard shade, it could be perfect for them.

As our single mother worked day and night to raise us, we saw firsthand how, against all odds in that day and age, she made her girls feel loved and encouraged and made them believe in themselves enough to do whatever they set out to accomplish. A gifted commercial artist and professional illustrator, her "tools of the trade" were our toys. We played with her glitter, colorful pencils, and paint. Not all of it landed on paper— we considered them our cosmetics as well! She always supported our creative and performance ambitions, both literally and figuratively, trading her artistic services for dance classes for us. She also endured countless stage shows we'd put on in the living room, always the attentive audience, no matter how exhausted she was.

The importance of self-esteem was something our mother tried to instill in us because she struggled with it all her life. It didn't come easy to us either, but her infinite faith in us gave us the confidence to believe in ourselves, which has been a driving factor in our success. A feminist before the term existed, our mother was a role model for us and many others, proving that sisters really can do it for themselves!

Like most successful businesses, Manic Panic was conceived as a solution to a problem. The idea to start our own business came from seeing the reaction people had to our trendsetting looks whenever we were out in clubs and onstage. The hip downtown crowd loved our unique punk style and wanted a place where they could buy it. Working for someone else had never really appealed to us, but we did need "day jobs" to supplement our love of the nightlife and our singing careers. Running a boutique that catered to rock and rollers and artists meant we didn't need to start work until somewhere around noon. There was a fashion void, and we were the right gals to fill it. We knew the underground culture because we were a part of it. NYC's East Village was the perfect location; it was the epicenter of punk. The city was almost bankrupt; there were lots of empty stores, and rent was dirt cheap!

So, along with our friend Gina Franklyn, we opened the only punk rock store in America, which was hailed by the press as the first of its kind. Soon, word of mouth spread, fans flocked, and rockers and celebrities donned their best disguises to rummage through racks of distinctive clothing (some we made ourselves), vintage stiletto shoes, fantasy hair color, cosmetics, and one-of-a-kind accessories.

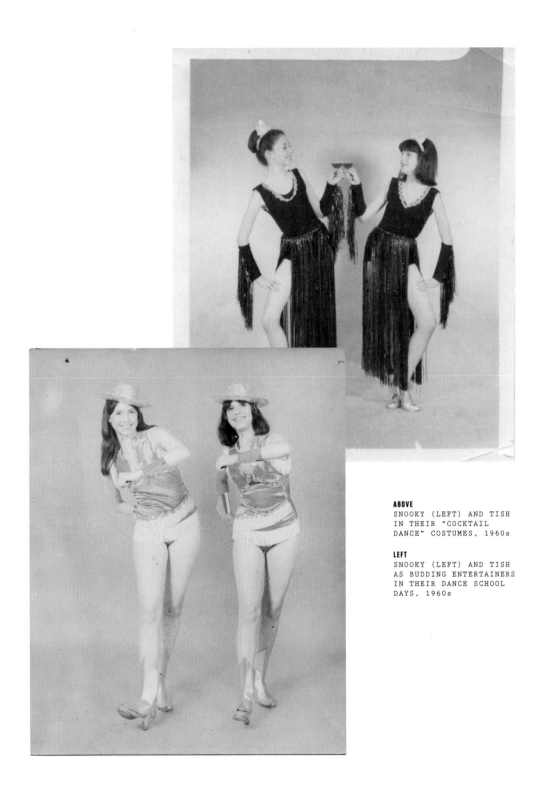

ABOVE
SNOOKY (LEFT) AND TISH
IN THEIR "COCKTAIL
DANCE" COSTUMES, 1960s

LEFT
SNOOKY (LEFT) AND TISH
AS BUDDING ENTERTAINERS
IN THEIR DANCE SCHOOL
DAYS, 1960s

I CAN'T THINK OF ANY BETTER REPRESENTATION OF BEAUTY THAN SOMEONE WHO IS UNAFRAID TO BE HERSELF.

—EMMA STONE

Accidental entrepreneurs, we didn't know what lay ahead of us. Although we had always dreamed of creating the world's first alternative beauty line, we never envisioned it would become what it is today. When we first started Manic Panic, there were hardly any independent beauty companies, and certainly not many owned by women, and definitely none that produced, created, and conceptualized like we did. We were just doing what had always served us best: following our instincts, making something out of nothing, and being badass, independent girls doing what we loved.

Ever since we opened our doors in 1977, Manic Panic has always been a safe haven for outsiders like us, from drag queens and club kids to performers and musicians and everyone who dares to be different. Through them, their feedback, and our own years onstage, we've learned the importance of high-quality, long-lasting, vibrant makeup and hair products, and so have our legions of fans. That's the magic of Manic Panic. There's a product and color for everyone, regardless of lifestyle and background!

Over the years, countless people have told us how coloring their hair with Manic Panic has made them feel visible and given them a surge of self-confidence, allowing them to show the world their inner sparkle! One story especially dear to us is from a woman named Rose, who was in her eighties when she first colored her hair purple. She said that before she colored her hair,

she felt invisible and nobody noticed or really cared to talk to her. Manic Panic Purple Haze was the gateway to her renaissance. People wanted to talk to "Purple Rose," interact with her, take pictures with her. She even wrote a poem about Manic Panic! This bold step made her so happy in the later years of her life. When she passed away, everyone attending her service paid tribute to her by wearing purple hair.

Living in Color not only tells our story but also gives you tools and hopefully inspires you to fearlessly celebrate your own unique beauty. We've always believed in expressing who we are, even when it was unfashionable or even dangerous to do so. With the mainstreaming of alternative beauty and a more personalized approach to self-expression these days, there has never been a better time to simply be yourself and live unapologetically and colorfully.

"Be who you are" doesn't mean being what the beauty industry dictates is "you," even if it's telling you that the trend is now to have blue hair. While we always advocate expressing your inner aurora borealis, it really doesn't matter if your hair is purple, green, pink, or even (gasp!) a natural color! Whatever's inside your heart and soul will shine through—all the rest is ephemeral.

To us, beauty isn't something that can be defined by one thing, one look, or one type. Beauty is found inside and out, and the most stunning people in the world are the ones who are truly themselves.

HAIR COLOR AND YOUR IDENTITY

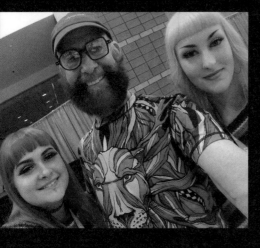

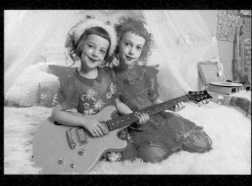

LEFT
MERMAID PARADE FIXTURE TODD KANE ROCKS A
RAINBOW BEARD USING SUNSHINE, WILDFIRE, ELECTRIC
LIZARD, ATOMIC TURQUOISE, AND ULTRA VIOLET.

ABOVE
OUR TINIEST BRAND AMBASSADORS, NAOMI AND ANNI
OF TINY BANGS, WEAR LIE LOCKS & CLEO ROSE AND
ATOMIC TURQUOISE, RESPECTIVELY, COURTESY OF
THEIR MOM, KIRSTEN.

We often hear from even the most seemingly conservative people that they used Manic Panic in their high school or college days. It's quite understandable that during such a tumultuous time in every young person's life, when we are trying to find where we fit in this world, Manic Panic would be a great coping mechanism.

"Hair may seem like a superfluous aspect of appearance, but studies show that our hair plays a central role in our identity, how we regard ourselves, as well as how we imagine we look to others," explains Tara Wells, a motivational psychologist and professor at Barnard College. "Having control over this aspect of our appearance and liking how our hair looks is integral to our overall self-confidence and self-esteem. A change in hair color may seem superficial, but it can signify a massive transformation happening within. Changing one's hair color can be a way of changing the game by giving you more confidence and the boost in self-esteem that comes from self-expression. A major change in appearance like hair color can signify starting a new chapter in life. For instance, after a breakup or changing jobs, it can send a message to the world that we are turning over a new leaf, starting a chapter, reinventing ourselves yet again."

DENNIS DUNAWAY,
FOUNDING MEMBER OF THE ALICE COOPER GROUP
AND ROCK AND ROLL HALL OF FAME INDUCTEE,
AND CURRENT MEMBER OF BLUE COUPE

Tish and Snooky are the outlandish legends of the New York City punk movement. The colorful sisters light up any room just by walking in, and their tight vocals and charismatic stage presence have earned them the endearing title of

"DARLINGS OF THE DEMENTED."

Their musical background is an amazing maze of interesting tales involving everyone who was anyone from CBGB and Max's Kansas City to their pioneering Manic Panic punk shop at Saint Marks Place. And now they've taken their punk look to the world and their colorful stories continue to unfold. When they walk into a room, it's as if someone has turned on a spotlight as people surround them for a closer look. Tish and Snooky's history is a fun inside look at the history of the New York scene. Everybody wants to be a part of their world, and now, finally, they're sharing their wonderful tales of underground glory.

THE 1970s:
THE BIRTH OF PUNK ROCK AND MANIC PANIC

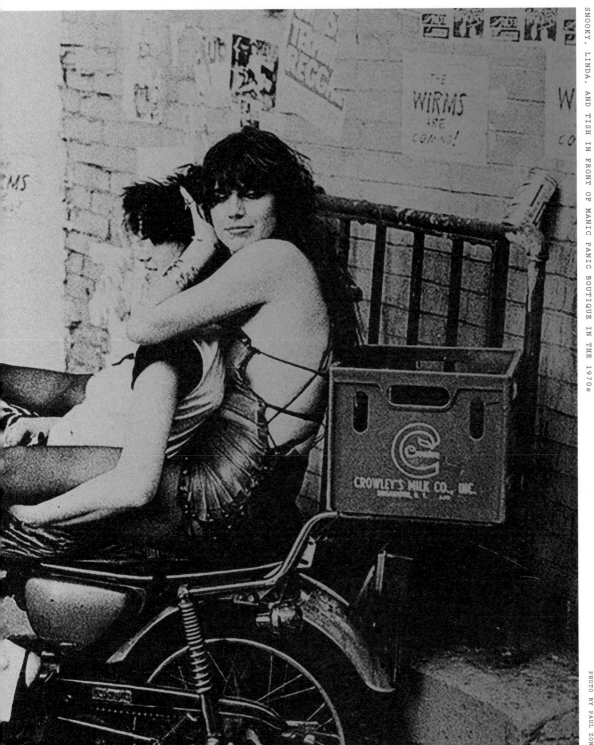

PHOTO BY PAUL ZONE

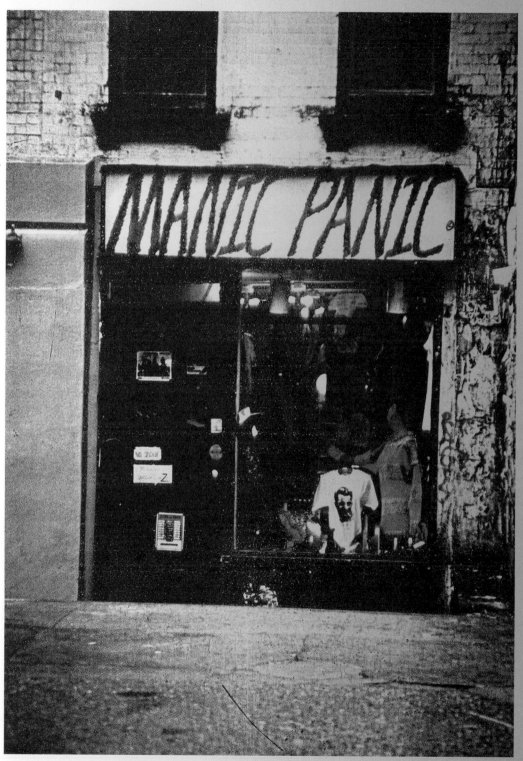

ORIGINAL MANIC PANIC STOREFRONT ON ST. MARKS PLACE, C. 1977
NOTICE THE COPYRIGHT SYMBOL ON THE SIGN. THAT'S A JEAN MICHEL BASQUIAT ORIGINAL! WE SCRAPED
OFF HIS ICONIC SIGNATURE "SAMO" AFTER HE GRAFITTIED OUR SIGN. OOPS!

THESE SISTERS HAVE MORE INNATE SPONTANEOUS STYLE IN THEIR PINKIES THAN MOST PEOPLE GOT IN THEIR LUMBERING CORPUSES.

—LESTER BANGS

Unless you were there, it's easy to glamorize New York City during the late 1970s as some sort of Technicolor dreamland filled with the best art, music, fashion, and beauty looks that have memorialized that decade. In reality, however, the city was often a rather unglamorous place, one that was crime-ridden, bankrupt, and grimy. Many of its residents were living in poverty and violence. Racism, drug abuse, and homophobia were daily reminders of a city divided.

Yet at the same time, it was also a magical haven for many. Struggling artists, musicians, poets, stylists, and entrepreneurs left their oppressive hometowns for a city where they could create, survive, and thrive in the midst of all the chaos. Two sisters hailing from the Bronx did just that. Hustling their way downtown to make their mark, they would breathe color not only into an entire city but also into an entire generation.

Patrice "Tish" and Eileen "Snooky" Bellomo were born in Manhattan but grew up living all over New York with their single mom. They eventually landed in the Bronx and started taking the subway to the clubs in lower Manhattan during the '70s, often "putting on their faces" during the hour-long train ride downtown.

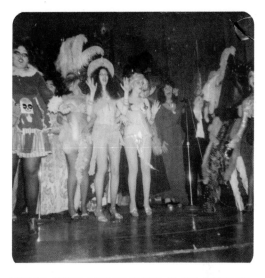

LEFT TO RIGHT: FAYETTE HAUSER OF THE COCKETTES, SNOOKY, TISH, AND WARHOL STAR MARIO MONTEZ (IN GREEN) ONSTAGE, PALM CASINO REVUE, 1974

"We were performing at a wacky, off-the-wall show across from CBGB," Tish recalls of their early days.

"Between shows, we'd run across the Bowery in our skimpy 'showgirl' costumes, which were actually recycled dance school costumes, minus the tutus, from our junior high school days. Traffic would stop! We'd do a quick guest appearance with Andy Warhol star Eric Emerson and the Magic Tramps, and then run back for the second show.

"Glamour was always much more important than warmth, and we'd never be dressed appropriately, especially in winter. On the coldest winter nights

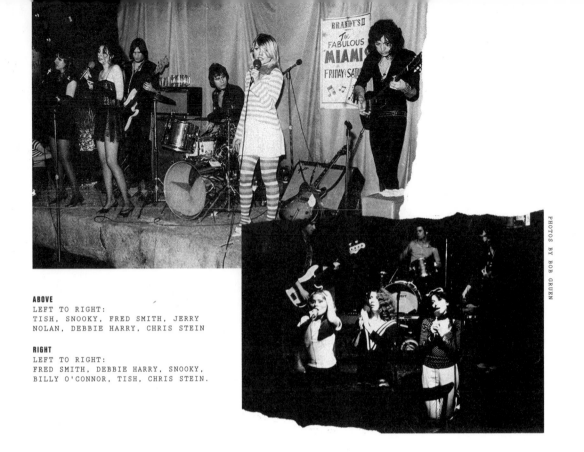

ABOVE
LEFT TO RIGHT:
TISH, SNOOKY, FRED SMITH, JERRY
NOLAN, DEBBIE HARRY, CHRIS STEIN

RIGHT
LEFT TO RIGHT:
FRED SMITH, DEBBIE HARRY, SNOOKY,
BILLY O'CONNOR, TISH, CHRIS STEIN.

we'd often be in tight sequined dresses, fishnets, spike-heeled shoes, and tiny jackets. 'Hathead' was never an option. One frigid night, we were on our way from CBGB to the 82 Club with our friend Joyce Francis, who went on to become a fashion designer/acrylic artist whose work can be seen in the Victoria and Albert Museum in London. We stopped in the vestibule of Phoebe's, one of the only restaurants on the Bowery at the time, in order to get warm before continuing on to the 82. The manager of the restaurant came out and said to us, 'LADIES! MY business isn't YOUR business, IF you know what I mean...' We had no idea what he meant, and said innocently, 'No, we don't know what you mean...' He repeated it again and told us we needed to move on. It dawned on us later that he thought we were, what was

called in those days, streetwalkers!"

Their big break came when Debbie Harry and Chris Stein came to see them perform. "Tomata du Plenty and Gorilla Rose, our friends in the show, had told Debbie and Chris that we'd be the perfect backup singers for Blondie, so they came to the show to see us," Snooky says. After joining a rehearsal for the new wave/punk band, they were hired.

"This was the first real downtown band we were ever in, so it was a big deal for us," Tish says. "The punk scene at the time was a really small, insular community. Back then everyone knew each other, so we'd be each other's audiences, fans, and critics.

"CBGB and Max's Kansas City were clubs where bands could actually perform original music—there were no cover bands allowed!"

YOU ARE CORDIALLY NOT INVITED!

"Our drummer at the time sometimes fell asleep in the dressing room between shows or missed gigs, so Jerry Nolan, the drummer of the New York Dolls, would be kind enough sit in for him. One night after a gig, he needed a ride to a fancy-pants party in Westchester. We crammed ourselves into 'The Blondie-mobile,' Debbie's 1967 Camaro. With Debbie at the wheel, along with Jerry Nolan, Chris Stein, Jimmy [from the Miamis] Wynbrandt, a boyfriend, and us, we drove off into the night to a party that we recall was hosted by some record company executive. Jerry was the only one actually invited, but we were all hell-bent on crashing the party! The car fit four comfortably, and there were six or seven of us. When we got to the house after a more-than-uncomfortable ride, the host would only allow Jerry in. We lurked outside, peering in the windows to see all of the most famous rock stars of the '70s enjoying the party. 'Look! There's Rod Stewart! Oh my God, is that Robert Plant?!' Soon Debbie and Chris managed to talk their way in. As the party was ending and guests were walking out, we weaseled our way in, much to the annoyance of the host. Today, if we could apologize to him we would, but we have no idea who he was! Sorry, dude!

"While managing the New York Dolls, Malcolm McLaren came to one of our gigs, and after the show we all went to the 210 Club, Harold Black's after-hours joint. Malcolm insisted that Blondie was a rotten name and that we'd never make it. He said 'Sex is a way better name for a band.' He went on to manage the Sex Pistols, and Blondie went on to the Rock and Roll Hall of Fame."

TOP RIGHT
BLONDIE AND THE BANZAI BABIES' ORIGINAL FLYER BY CHRIS STEIN, LIVE AT HILLY'S (AKA CBGB), C. 1975

BOTTOM RIGHT
BATHROOM WALL AT CBGB WITH TISH AND SNOOKY GRAFFITI (NOT WRITTEN BY THEM)

During this time, fashion and beauty trends in the city were morphing, somewhere between glam and punk. It was an awkward phase when everybody was experimenting with various looks. The sisters were scoring their clothing at thrift shops, junk stores, and dumpsters. They were throwing things together and sewing up fashion from scraps to make original outfits that looked great in dark clubs or onstage (although maybe less so up close).

"Debbie would take us to her favorite thrift shops in New Jersey and we'd all

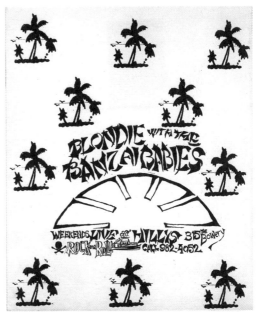

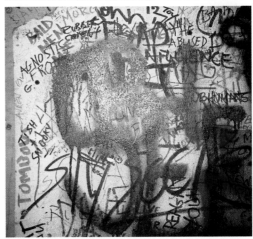

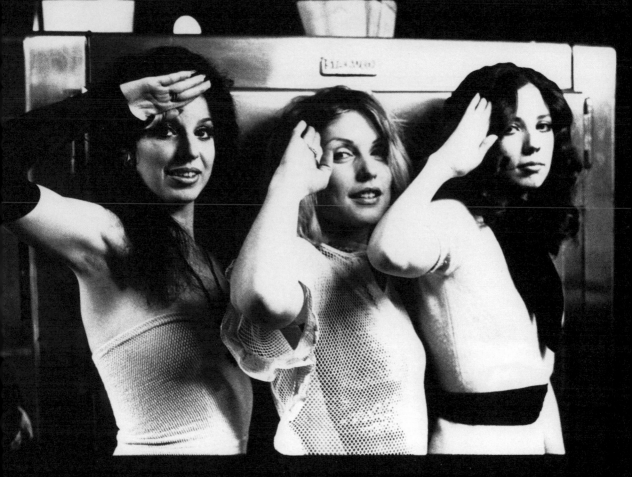

BLONDIE DAYS, C. 1975
(LEFT TO RIGHT: TISH BELLOMO, DEBBIE HARRY, SNOOKY BELLOMO)
PHOTO BY CHRIS STEIN

WE DO HAVE A LONG LIST OF PEOPLE THAT HELPED GET US HERE—AND SOME OF THEM ARE ACTUALLY PERFORMERS, AND SOME OF THEM ARE ACTUALLY GIRLS. SO, TISH AND SNOOKY...WHEREVER YOU MAY BE, THANK YOU FROM THE BOTTOM OF MY HEART.

—DEBBIE HARRY, ROCK AND ROLL HALL OF FAME INDUCTION SPEECH

find stuff to wear onstage," Snooky recalls. "And then we'd take her to the Bronx to our favorite thrift shops." Soon thereafter, their love of thrifting led to them throwing "rock 'n' roll rummage sales" with their friend Gina Franklyn, who had a loft on Second Avenue and St. Marks Place during the late '70s.

The loft sales basically served as a makeshift vintage pop-up for stuff they'd bring down from the Bronx, as well as rock 'n' roll memorabilia they were collecting.

"Somehow, probably through a trade, I acquired a scarf that had once belonged to Johnny Thunders of the New York Dolls, so that's how our first sale qualified as a 'rock 'n' roll' rummage sale. We were friends with the bands, as well as friends of friends of the bands, and trading was popular back then," Snooky says. "A friend of ours, Jimmy Wynbrandt from the band the Miamis (who opened for the New York Dolls at the infamous 82 Club), had come into possession of Johnny Thunders' beat-up old vintage black leather motorcycle jacket. I just had to have it! I traded it for a warm, fleece-lined brown bomber

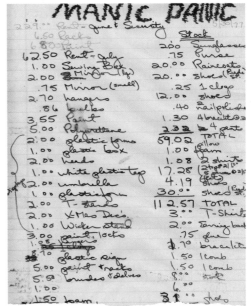

jacket that my boyfriend, rockabilly singer Robert Gordon, had given me. Boy, was he mad!" Snooky laughs. "I still have Johnny's jacket! It was even featured in a punk exhibit at the Museum of Sex in New York. In retrospect, I think I got the better end of the deal."

After hosting several of these sales, word of mouth spread quickly. Eventually, Tish, Snooky, and Gina decided to open a shop of their own, where they could sell whatever they wanted co-op style—everything from original designs and imports to hair color, cosmetics, and unused vintage. Since Gina's place was nearby, they looked around St. Marks Place, which at the time was littered with ex-hippies, junkies, and, most importantly, empty storefronts. The rent was cheap and the neighborhood was familiar, so they signed a lease on the spot.

After many rejected store name ideas, such as Band Aid and the Walking Wounded, their mother, who worked in a psychiatric hospital as an art therapist, suggested Manic Panic, a term used to describe a state experienced by manic

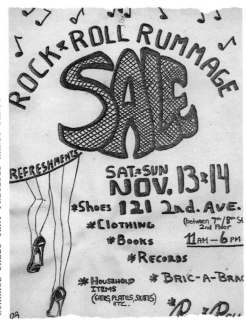

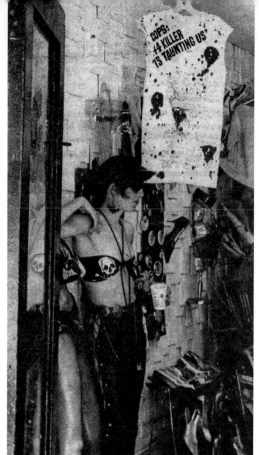

COPS: '4 KILLER 'IS TAUNTING US'

THERE IS NO EXQUISITE BEAUTY WITHOUT SOME STRANGENESS IN THE PROPORTION.

—EDGAR ALLAN POE

depressives. The minute the girls heard it, they knew it had the perfect badass attitude, the exact mood they wanted the store to exude. Tish designed the logo and hand-painted the plastic light box sign above the store window. Soon enough, the slightly controversial two-word phrase became not just a store but a brand synonymous with all things punk rock.

Along with the arsenal of punk rock goods, sharkskin suits from the '50s and '60s (some with their original tags—Elvis Costello bought a couple!), unused Beatle boots, and "Spring-o-lator" stiletto shoes, Tish and Gina made and designed original clothing, T-shirts, and accessories, including Tish's hand-painted Son of Sam T-shirts and Snooky-knitted sweaters. She had an amazing eye for

finding cool vintage items—all completely unused! They both defaced old David Cassidy and Farrah Fawcett T-shirts with punk slogans and cigarette burns.

They dumpster-dove at night for store fixtures and mannequins in the garbage. It was behind the department store where Snooky had been working, but the store was going out of business at the time. They still have some of those mannequins to this day! Manic Panic, the first-ever punk store in America, was ready to rock!

And maniacal it was: On the day of the official store opening and official press reception—July 7, 1977, or 7/7/77— they received a ton of publicity, and soon after, every major TV network and newspaper in the country featured the unusual little shop. "I think this auspicious date was suggested by our friend and customer,

Manic Panic was our

UNOFFICIAL HEADQUARTERS

in the Dead Boys' earliest days in NYC. Our days began in the early afternoon, and we would hit Stromboli's for pizza, Gem Spa for cigarettes, and Manic Panic to see what Tish and Snooky had come up with and hang out. Manic Panic was as much our headquarters as CBGB was!

—CHEETAH CHROME, DEAD BOYS

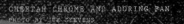

writer Toby Goldstein," Snooky recalls. "We didn't even know what a press reception was, but she helped us. We invited all the press, media people, and local punk bands (members of the Ramones, the Dictators, the Dead Boys, etc.) that we all knew."

More music icons such as Richard Hell (who originated the iconic punk spiked haircut), the Cramps, the B-52's, and the Stranglers were soon seen roaming the store, stocking up on new looks. Tish remembers, "Patti Smith would drop by with copies of her latest poetry for us to sell to 'help pay the 'lectric bill.'" Debbie Harry was kind enough to do a photo shoot right in the store window, modeling Manic Panic fashions. Manic Panic had become the ultimate pit stop for punk rockers in New York City.

Early Manic Panic employee Joe Katz remembers helping customers from the Buzzcocks to Caroline Kennedy: "Robert Fripp was a weekly pinball contest winner on our beat-up machine. Mick Jagger and Jerry Hall even stopped by!" The unconventional clothing, accessories, and beauty products they carried helped bands find their own unique look and style, leading to more exposure for themselves as well as the store.

Sensing that the phenomenon they had just ignited could grow, Tish, Snooky,

and Gina started traveling to London with suitcases full of American goods to sell, like cool sunglasses, deadstock dresses from the '60s, and stiletto shoes from the '50s. But the girls also scoped out what sort of things England had to offer, fashion- and beauty-wise. "We'd shop all day and go to the clubs and shows all night. Gina's brother gave us a room over his pub or else we'd stay at a squat on Lots Road that our friend 'Billy Boop' shared with other squatters. It was an abandoned house, we slept on the floor, there was no heat, electricity, or indoor plumbing, so it was a big production to go downstairs to the outhouse. It was dangerous to go outside alone, so we'd all go downstairs together, en masse, lighting our way with a candle. And it was sooooo cooooold! But it was worth it. When we told the toothless old man working at the neighborhood fish and chips shop exactly where we were staying, he said in absolute disgust, 'Oh! I know them stinky little houses!'"

On one of their first trips to the UK, they realized a big opportunity was vibrant, unnatural hair color, a relatively unknown product in the United States. The girls arrived with offerings from America, sold everything in their suitcases, and then filled them back up with a carefully curated selection of hair colors, vinyl records, fanzines, and other "contraband" from London to resell at Manic Panic. Gina was British, so she knew a lot about the punk scene there and knew where to shop. Snooky says, "We were cross-pollinating! We'd go to Vivienne Westwood's store, Seditionaries, and buy loads of outrageous and controversial T-shirts. One time Vivienne herself helped me with my purchase, kindly offering to make me a dummy invoice at a much lower price so I wouldn't have to pay as much duty on it, not that we ever did anyway! We'd always just casually waltz through customs with 'nothing to declare.'"

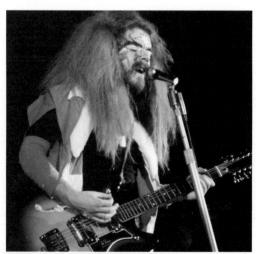

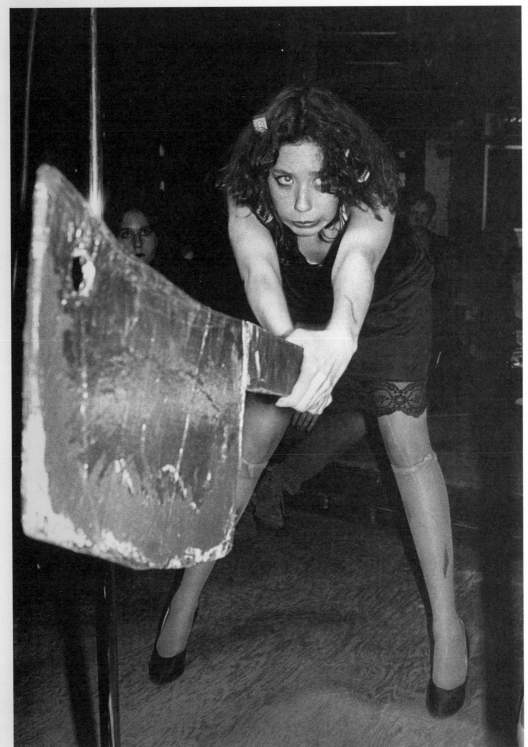

SNOOKY ONSTAGE WITH THE SIC F*CKS. "NO ONE CALLS ME ABSOLUTELY RIDICULOUS AND GETS AWAY WITH IT!"

PHOTO BY EBET ROBERTS

Before Manic Panic opened in New York City, the only people known for dyeing their hair in extreme colors were fearless artists like Roy Wood, David Bowie, Cherry Vanilla, and Todd Rundgren.

"Debbie Harry had told us that it had been a trend in her high school to color blond hair with food coloring, so she was probably one of the first to ever go pink," Tish says. However, food coloring usually washes right out, so with Manic Panic's introduction of their long-lasting, semi-permanent hair colors, wild looks became even more possible and shocking.

"I think you could call us pirates," Tish says with a laugh before Snooky chimes in, "Or international smugglers!" On one of these trips, a TSA agent asked the girls why they had so many hair colors in their bag. They batted their eyelashes and exclaimed, "Well, we wanted to try every color!"

The girls became walking advertisements for the unconventional dyes. Gina rocked short, choppy, Johnny Rotten-inspired orangey-red hair, while Tish's hair was dyed a dark fuchsia, but she'd let her roots grow out, bleach them, let her roots grow out again, and then bleach them again, creating "stripes" so she looked like her tabby cat, Waldo. Their hair generated lots of attention everywhere they went, sometimes provoking angry and even violent reactions.

"I went to the opening night of the Mudd Club," Tish reflects. "As I left and was trying to hail a cab, a bunch of nasty suburban guys pulled over, hopped out of their car, and started a street fight with us. I woke up to the siren screams of an ambulance. I had been sucker-punched in the face and knocked unconscious for about five minutes! In those days, punk fashions and brightly colored hair brought out hostility and anger in some people. They hated anyone who dared to be or look different."

"After visiting a friend dying in the hospital, I was walking dejectedly down

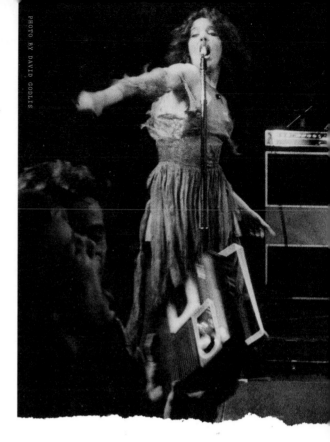

Fifth Avenue when a Rolls-Royce pulled up beside me," Snooky remembers. "The window opened, and a weaselly, little straight guy in a suit leaned out and screamed, 'Y'know, you look absolutely ridiculous! *ABSOLUTELY RIDICULOUS!*' before driving off, very proud of himself for publicly belittling me."

A quote we love, which has been attributed to Marilyn Monroe, although some say it wasn't really hers, sums it up perfectly:

"Imperfection is beauty, madness is genius, and it's better to be absolutely ridiculous than absolutely boring!"

While their look wasn't common, it was popular with the creative crowd. Their shop made a name for itself by supplying hair color in every shade of the rainbow, as well as rare beauty finds such as black lipstick and nail polish and face and body glitters. People of all ages, drag queens, punk rockers, and members of the LGBTQ+ community were flocking to Manic Panic's doors to

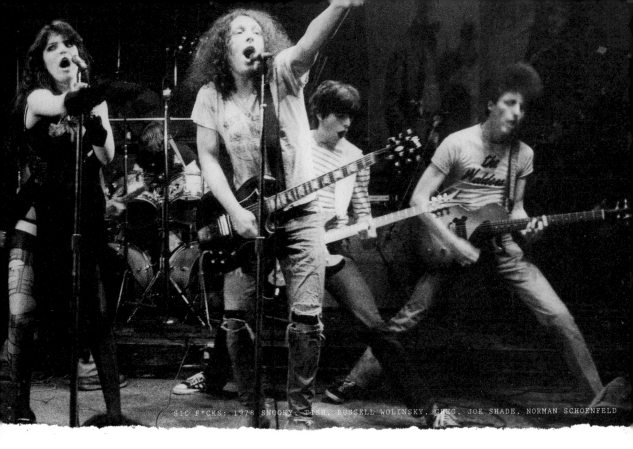

SIC F*CKS; 1978 SNOOKY, TISH, RUSSELL WOLINSKY, GREG, JOE SHADE, NORMAN SCHOENFELD

find both clothing and beauty products to express themselves more authentically and artistically. During the Halloween season, it became the hot spot in NYC with a line around the corner to get in. Everyone wanted to be a punk rocker for a day!

Gina had decided to leave less than a year after the store opening. "It must have been hard working with two sisters who thought so alike most of the time," says Tish. "She'd often be outvoted! Also, since she was English, she was more into the UK punk style and we were more into the NYC style." In addition to their St. Marks Place location, Hilly Kristal, owner of CBGB, had rented a little store in the CBGB Theater on Second Avenue to the three girls. Gina suggested she take the theater store and the sisters keep the store on St. Marks Place. So they parted ways amicably.

By the end of the '70s, Manic Panic was booming. The store had established

its own eccentric personality and had become the go-to place for everything from wigs, hair dye, and cosmetics to latex clothing, Mary Quant hosiery, and Doc Martens boots. Tish and Snooky worked nonstop: during the day at Manic Panic, and at night rocking out with their punk band, the Sic F*cks.

But hardships were looming, and Tish and Snooky were about to face their biggest challenges yet: Being poor, being women, and being new business owners meant dealing with an unpredictable economy and unrelenting discrimination, not to mention copycats and new competition capitalizing on their innovative style.

Times were changing almost as fast as Tish and Snooky changed their hair colors. With the 1980s approaching, it was time for them to put on their highest stiletto heels, tease up their big '80s hair, and stand tall against "the man"—or dye trying.

BEFORE THE RAINBOW,

THERE WAS BLACK OR BLOND

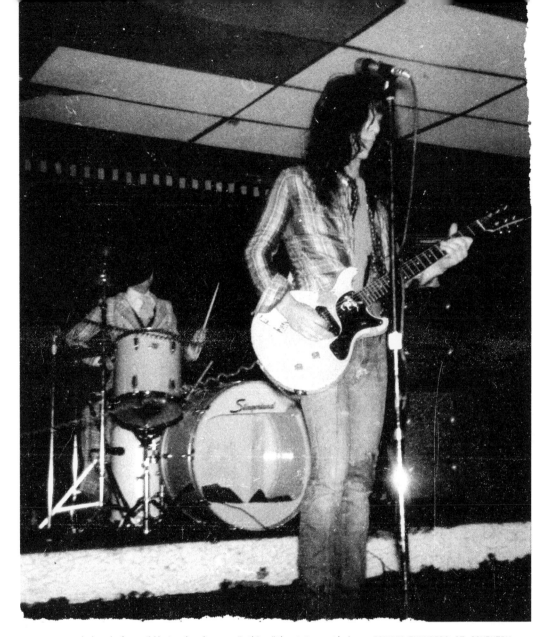

*I*n pre-punk days before wild hair colors became "a thing," the statement hair colors of choice for the most part were black and blond. Unnatural raven black and bleached blond hair have always been the epitome of cool. From Vampirella, Elvis, Johnny Thunders, and Alice Cooper on the dark side to Marilyn Monroe, Mary Weiss (lead singer of the Shangri-Las), and later Debbie Harry on the blond side, these were the two coolest hair colors of the time.

Of course, there was the eternally cool Lucille Ball's shade of unnatural red, which we always loved, but red was the exception to the rule—for the most part, in the early days, it was a black-and-white hair world.

Siouxsie Sioux's "Theda Bara Goes Goth" look and Joan Jett's signature shag, with Raven black hair and eyeshadow to match, is a punk classic.

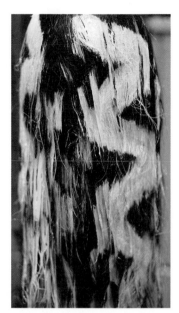

CREATING DESIGNS WITH BLEACH
IS EASY USING MANIC PANIC FLASH
LIGHTNING BLEACH.

I WANNA BE A PLATINUM BLOND!

Blond has always been glamorous, sexy, and cool. As punk's ultimate poster child, blond bombshell Debbie Harry said in Blondie's song "Platinum Blonde": "Marilyn and Jean, Jane, May and Marlene, they proved it, they really had fun!" But Debbie had her own unique take on blond. She'd leave the back part of her hair dark, which is the ultimate in cool—making no attempt to look like an actual natural blond. Today it's a big trend to have dark roots, but to Debbie, it was just her being herself. And bleach blond wasn't only for women. Men like Andy Warhol, Billy Idol, and John Sex are prime examples. David Bowie, Iggy Pop, and Lou Reed all went through their blond phases.

WHY PRE-LIGHTENING YOUR HAIR IS IMPORTANT

Although certain Manic Panic shades can be applied over natural hair colors and can give beautiful highlights, it's highly recommended to first prelighten your hair to achieve the best, most vibrant results and to get the most out of your chosen creative color. The removal of color is also known as *lift*, a word you'll see used when referring to bleaching and from stylists quoted in this book. Since natural, uncolored hair is smooth—and therefore not very porous or absorbent—bleaching (aka lightening) the hair first will make the hair light enough for the colors to really pop, and the bleach will activate and open the cuticles of the hair strands so that the dye molecules can fully saturate them.

When semi-permanent colors are applied to natural hair, the molecules can sometimes slide off the smooth surface when you rinse or wash your locks, which can result in a color that might fade more quickly. Even if you're a natural blonde and the color you apply is initially bold, it can typically fade much faster than it would on prelightened, porous hair.

For prelightening, natural blond hair might require a lower volume developer (which can range from 5 to 20 or higher volume), instead of the higher, more powerful volumes that dark and coarse hair might need (30–40 volume). As always, if you're unsure about what to use, consult with a stylist you trust beforehand.

As your hair grows out, if you're not a big fan of roots, you'll want to touch up the new growth before recoloring. When lightening the roots, be careful not to overlap on hair that has already been prelightened, as this can cause breakage and damage the hair.

★ HOT TIP

AFTER YOU LIGHTEN YOUR HAIR, WASH IT AT LEAST THREE TIMES TO GET ALL THE RESIDUE OFF. IF THERE IS STILL BLEACH IN YOUR HAIR, THE COLOR YOU THEN APPLY CAN SOMETIMES START FADING RIGHT BEFORE YOUR EYES!

MANIC PANIC® N.Y.C.

TISH & SNOOKY'S

100% CRUELTY-FREE & *Vegan* SEMI PERMANENT HAIR COLOR

HIGH VOLTAGE CLASSIC AND AMPLIFIED FORMULA

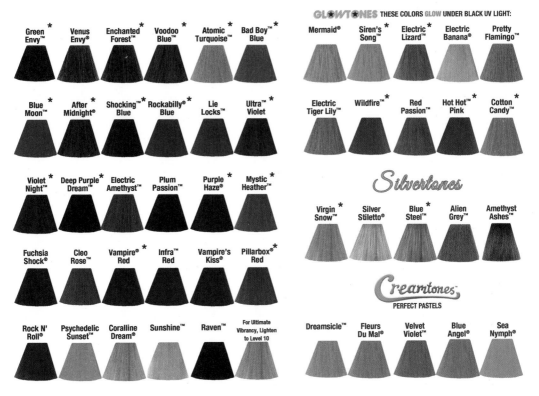

Green Envy™ * Venus Envy® Enchanted Forest™ * Voodoo Blue™ * Atomic Turquoise™ * Bad Boy™ Blue

Blue Moon™ * After Midnight® Shocking™ Blue Rockabilly® Blue Lie Locks™ Ultra™ Violet *

Violet Night™ * Deep Purple Dream™ * Electric Amethyst™ * Plum Passion™ Purple Haze® * Mystic Heather™ *

Fuchsia Shock® Cleo Rose™ Vampire® Red * Infra™ Red Vampire's Kiss® Pillarbox® Red

Rock N' Roll® Psychedelic Sunset™ Coralline Dream® Sunshine™ Raven™ For Ultimate Vibrancy, Lighten to Level 10

GLOWTONES THESE COLORS GLOW UNDER BLACK UV LIGHT:

Mermaid® Siren's Song™ * Electric Lizard™ * Electric Banana® Pretty Flamingo™

Electric Tiger Lily™ Wildfire™ * Red Passion™ Hot Hot™ Pink Cotton Candy™

Silvertones

Virgin Snow™ * Silver Stiletto® Blue Steel™ * Alien Grey™ Amethyst Ashes™

Creamtones™
PERFECT PASTELS

Dreamsicle™ Fleurs Du Mal® Velvet Violet™ Blue Angel® Sea Nymph®

*These colors are available in both the Classic and extra pigmented Amplified Formulas. Coralline Dream is only available in Amplified.

TISH & SNOOKY'S®

MANIC PANIC®
N.Y.C.
PROFESSIONAL

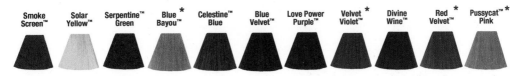

Smoke Screen™ Solar Yellow™ Serpentine™ Green Blue Bayou™ * Celestine™ Blue Blue Velvet™ Love Power Purple™ Velvet Violet™ * Divine Wine™ Red Velvet™ * Pussycat™ Pink *

*These colors glow under black UV light.

ALL THE COLORS OF THE MANIC PANIC RAINBOW!

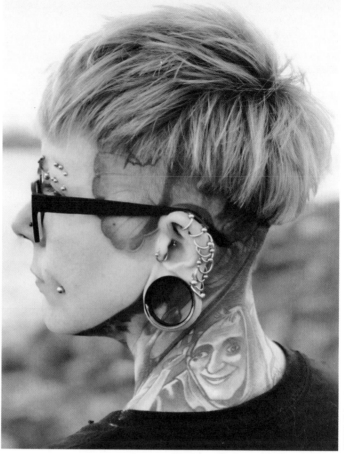

PHOTO BY NICO NORRIS

Before applying any Manic Panic color, we recommend that you prelighten your hair to a level 9 or higher for the most vibrant results. Darker and warmer shades can work well on hair that's been lifted to a medium blond, or a level 6. A level 10 platinum blond is required for pastel shades, like Creamtones or any shades you may want to make lighter yourself using our Pastel-izer, as well as for platinums, silvers, and grays, such as Alien Grey, Amethyst Ashes, Blue Steel, Silver Stiletto, and Virgin Snow.

LIGHTENING PERMANENTLY DYED HAIR

Don't try this at home! Do not apply bleach to hair already dyed with a permanent hair color, even if it's a shade of blond. Many contain metallic salts that can be extremely damaging when combined with bleach and can cause the hair to break off completely. If you want to bleach hair that's been permanently dyed, consult with a professional hair colorist first, so they can evaluate the current condition of your hair.

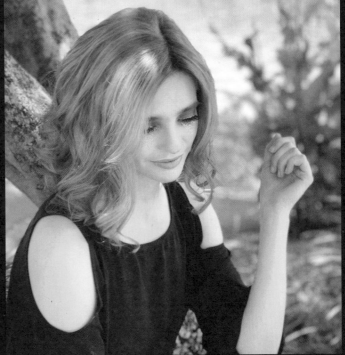

A SMOKY RAINBOW CREATED BY STYLIST CHELSEA MANFRE FOR OUR 2018 BRUSHES UP CONTEST AT PREMIERE ORLANDO

PHOTO BY CHELSEA MANFRE

HOW TO AVOID OVERBLEACHING AND DAMAGING YOUR HAIR

If you have undergone multiple chemical processes, such as permanent waves, permanent color, or lightening, your hair can take many years to completely grow out and attain its full strength, as the average person's hair grows at ¼ inch a month. Covering damage with a darker color can hide it, but the abuse is still there.

If you insist on attempting to bleach previously treated hair (and don't say we didn't warn ya!), it is imperative to do a strand test. Take a small section toward the back of the hair, using foil or another material to separate it from the rest of the hair. Apply the bleach to the strand and check it at ten-minute intervals, being sure to pull the ends of your hair between two fingers. If any hair resembles ramen noodles and has broken off, it is time to rinse immediately. Remember that as long as hair is wet, it will continue to process! Even though water will decelerate the rate at which the hair is lifting, it will not stop until you shampoo your hair a few times.

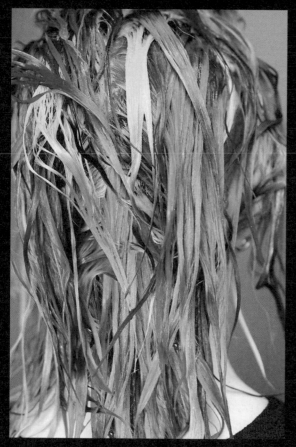

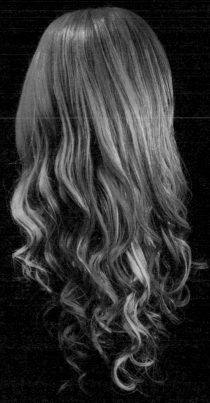

HOW TO COLOR YOUR HAIR USING MANIC PANIC

Always begin with a test strand on a small section of hair that is some-what hidden on your head but easy to reach, following the steps for coloring on page 37. Once you are happy with the color on your test, follow these steps to achieve the raddest and most badass hair color at home!

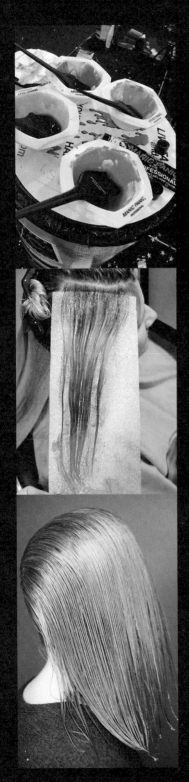

1. IF YOU HAVEN'T JUST PRELIGHTENED YOUR HAIR, FIRST WASH THE HAIR WITH A DEEP CLEANSING OR CLARIFYING SHAMPOO, PREFERABLY ONE WITHOUT SULFATES. DO NOT FOLLOW UP WITH ANY CONDITIONER.

2. NEXT, DRY THE HAIR TO REMOVE EXCESS WATER AND ENSURE THAT THE HAIR IS EXTREMELY POROUS BEFORE COLORING.

3. APPLY A THIN LAYER OF PETROLEUM JELLY AROUND THE HAIRLINE AND ON EARS TO AVOID DYEING YOUR SKIN. PLEASE MAKE SURE YOU'RE WEARING PLASTIC GLOVES, EVEN WHEN WORKING WITH LIGHTER COLORS, TO GUARANTEE THAT THERE WON'T BE ANY HAIR DYE STAINS TRANSFERRED TO YOUR SKIN OR OTHER SURFACES.

4. TIME FOR THE FUN PART—THE MANIC PANIC COLOR APPLICATION! USING A TINT BRUSH OR YOUR GLOVED FINGERS, BEGIN APPLYING COLOR IN SMALL SECTIONS, STARTING AT THE ROOTS AND WORKING YOUR WAY DOWN THROUGH TO THE ENDS OF THE HAIR.

5. ONCE YOU'VE APPLIED THE MANIC PANIC COLOR ONTO THE DESIRED AREAS OF THE HAIR, COMB THROUGH THE HAIR COLOR TO MAKE SURE IT IS EVENLY APPLIED AND THE HAIR IS THOROUGHLY SATURATED THROUGHOUT. NOTE: DON'T FRET IF THE HAIR DYE BECOMES SLIGHTLY FROTHY. THIS IS NORMAL!

6. NOW, SIMPLY COVER COLORED HAIR WITH A PLASTIC CAP.

7. IF YOU LIKE, YOU CAN REMOVE THE CAP AND USE A HAIR DRYER TO APPLY HEAT FOR PART OF THE PROCESSING TIME. THIS WILL HELP OPEN UP THE HAIR CUTICLES AND ALLOW THE MANIC PANIC HAIR COLOR TO BETTER PENETRATE THE HAIR STRANDS FOR OPTIMUM COLOR PAYOFF. PUT THE CAP BACK ON.

8. LEAVE COLOR ON FOR THIRTY TO FORTY-FIVE MINUTES, AND SIT BACK, RELAX, AND DREAM OF THE AMAZING NEW HAIR COLOR THAT'S BREWING!

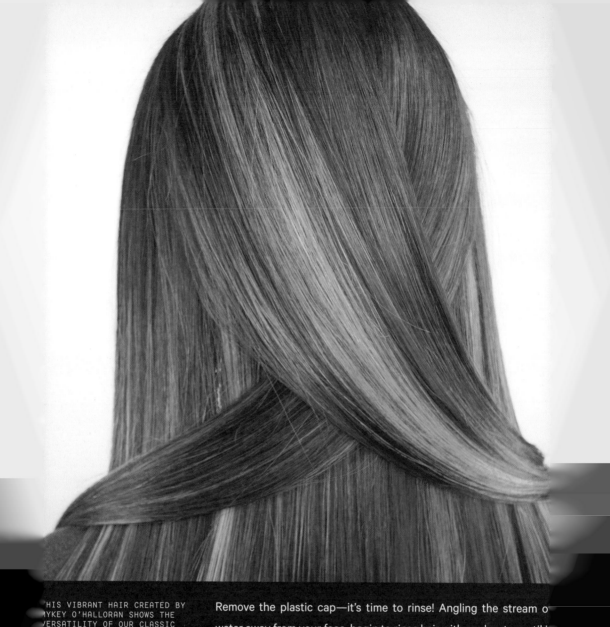

Remove the plastic cap—it's time to rinse! Angling the stream of water away from your face, begin to rinse hair with cool water until it runs clear and there's no longer any color washing rinsing off. Do not use shampoo or conditioner when rinsing.

Don't worry if at first glance your wet hair isn't the color you imagined. You can't really tell the true shade until it is completely dry. Towel and/or blow-dry your hair to see your final results and style as usual.

Voilà! You are now ready for your close-up! Blast your favorite song ("She's a Rainbow" by the Rolling Stones is always apropos) while flipping your fabulous new hair side to side with your cell on slo-mo!

TRICKS FOR MAKING YOUR COLOR LAST LONGER

A helpful tip for making your hair color last longer is to rinse the hair with a mixture of vinegar and water immediately after coloring. This technique balances the pH level of the hair, which gives it more permanence.

Here's a simple step-by-step:

1. RINSE OUT THE MANIC PANIC COLOR WITH COOL WATER UNTIL YOUR HAIR IS FREE OF DYE AND THE WATER RUNS CLEAR.

2. MIX A SMALL AMOUNT OF WHITE OR APPLE CIDER VINEGAR WITH WATER, AND POUR THE MIXTURE DIRECTLY OVER THE HAIR.

3. GENTLY COMB THROUGH THE HAIR AND LET IT SIT FOR A COUPLE OF MINUTES.

4. RINSE OUT WITH COLD WATER, BEING SURE TO AVOID GETTING ANY IN YOUR EYES.

Another way to make sure your chosen shade stays as vivid and healthy as possible is to wash semi-regularly with a sulfate-free, color-safe shampoo and conditioner using cool water only. The more you wash the hair, the faster the color will fade, so try to wash as infrequently as possible.

To minimize the amount of times you wash your hair, try applying a dry shampoo in between regular shampoos. You can also mix in any leftover hair color into your conditioner after shampooing for optimal hair color maintenance.

RED,
THE
GATEWAY
TO BOLD

COLOR GUIDE

MANIC PANIC CLASSIC HIGH VOLTAGE, AMPLIFIED, AND PROFESSIONAL COLORS

| INFRA RED | PILLARBOX RED | RED PASSION | ROCK 'N' ROLL RED | WILDFIRE | VAMPIRE RED | RED VELVET | DIVINE WINE |

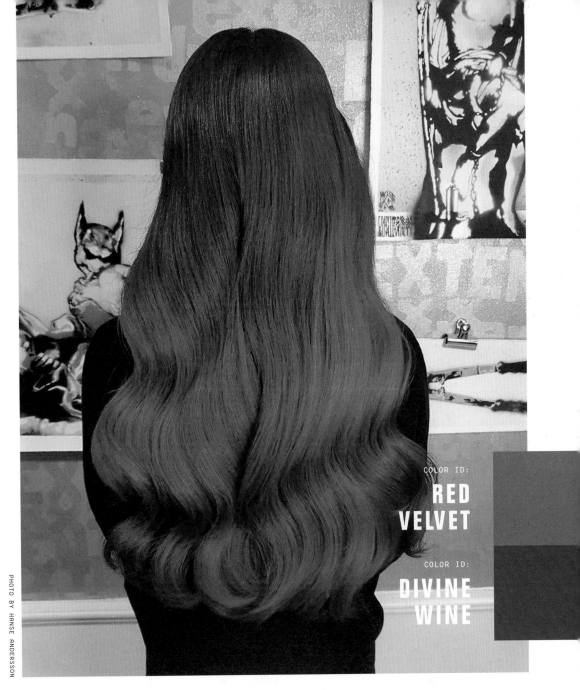

COLOR ID:

RED VELVET

COLOR ID:

DIVINE WINE

HANSE ANDERSSON MAKES RED LOOK RAVISHING WITH A RED VELVET AND DIVINE WINE BLEND.

n the 1970s, punk rockers like Nina Hagen, Johnny Rotten, and Cherry Vanilla were some of the first rocking redheads to venture into the colorful world of unnatural hair dye, while Poison Ivy of the Cramps rocked beautiful, natural red hair. Fans who saw them hanging out at CBGB or in the back room of Max's Kansas City copied their look, so red hair dye was one of the first colors to really take off at Manic Panic.

★ 43

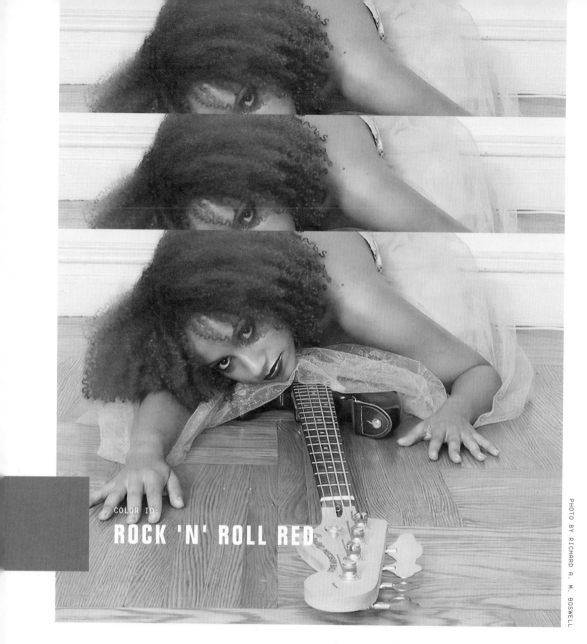

COLOR ID:

ROCK 'N' ROLL RED

THE INCREDIBLE
MILITIA VOX IN
ROCK 'N' ROLL RED.

Red was Snooky's "gateway" hair color as well. "I first started out with a more natural shade of red, then graduated to bright red stripes a la Bride of Frankenstein. Then, as time went on, it got more and more vibrant, in-your-face, outrageous, and obnoxious," she says with a laugh. "It's a totally F-you color that I proudly wore for years. I loved that it made some people so mad!"

Johnny Rotten had bright orange/red hair during the Sex Pistols' final tour in 1978. He later said in an interview,

"I LOVE DISCORDANCY.

It makes people ill at ease and wakes up a part of their brain that's normally asleep. It's nice to be irritated."

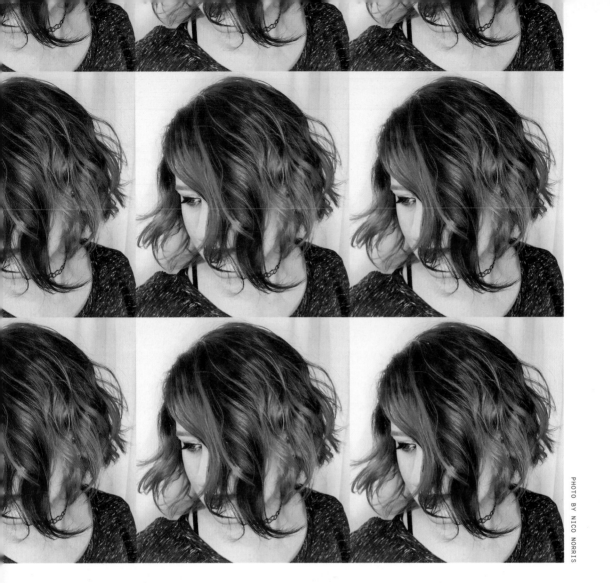

BRAND AMBASSADOR NICO NORRIS CREATES A BLAZE OF RED USING CUSTOM BLENDS OF LOVE POWER PURPLE, DEEP PURPLE DREAM, PLUM PASSION, RED VELVET, BLUE VELVET, SOLAR YELLOW, INFRA RED, SMOKESCREEN, AND RAVEN.

High-vibe hair color beautician Roxie Darling agrees and has some advice for beginners: "Red is the hardest hair color to keep, and also the hardest hair color to get rid of. I recommend making sure you *really* want to go red before you dye it. When it comes to skin tone, whatever color you choose will be projecting itself onto your face, so think about basic color theory and how colors interact with one another and how the color you are adding to your hair will mix with the color of your skin tone."

She also notes, "It's really important to get clear on the exact red that you want to be: Do you want it to be more of a classic red with warm undertones, like orange or copper? If so, you'll want to grab Manic Panic's Pillarbox Red and Vampire Red, which you could even mix with some Psychedelic Sunset to achieve those rich warm undertones. Or, do you want something on the deeper side that is more of a blue-hued red? If so, I recommend mixing Red Passion and Vampire Red with a tiny drop of Purple Haze to add some depth."

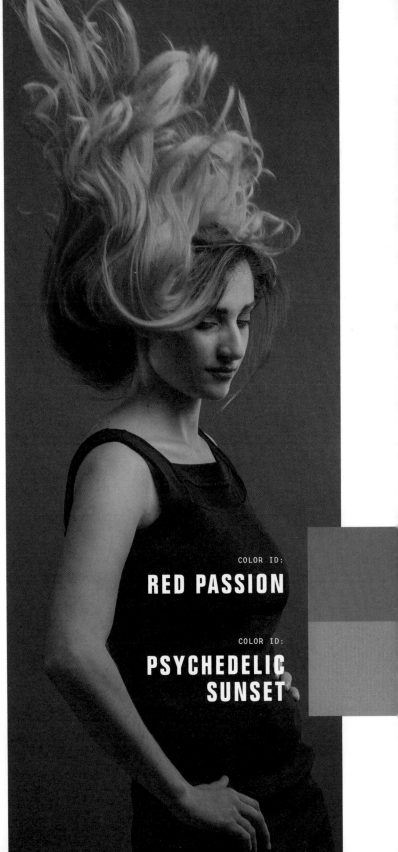

PHOTO BY KEREN BENISTI

KEREN BENISTI
CREATED THIS
FLAMING-RED HAIRDO
USING RED PASSION
AND PSYCHEDELIC
SUNSET.

COLOR ID:

RED PASSION

COLOR ID:

**PSYCHEDELIC
SUNSET**

GREEN

WITH (VENUS) ENVY

COLOR GUIDE

ELECTRIC LIZARD	ENCHANTED FOREST	GREEN ENVY	SIREN'S SONG	VENUS ENVY	SERPENTINE GREEN

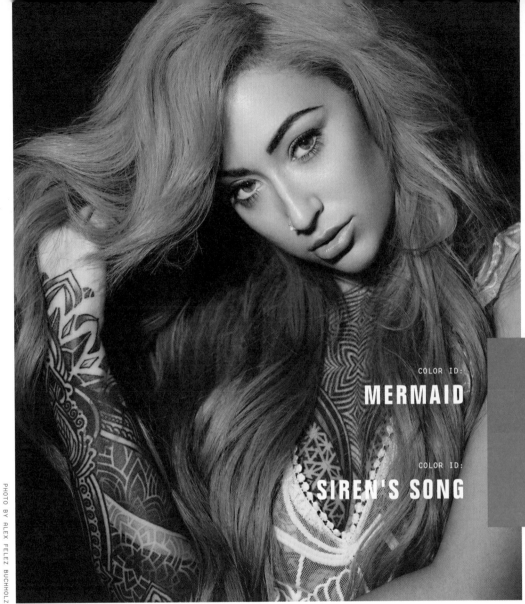

COLOR ID:

MERMAID

COLOR ID:

SIREN'S SONG

G reen was also big in the '70s, a favorite of Mohawk-sporting punks, as well as Todd Rundgren, who for a time dyed his long hair green, as did teenage Nick Berlin from the Blessed and Poly Styrene from X-Ray Spex.

MODEL SUMMER McINERNEY ROCKS A GORGEOUS MONOCHROMATIC GREEN MANE MIXING MERMAID AND SIREN'S SONG.

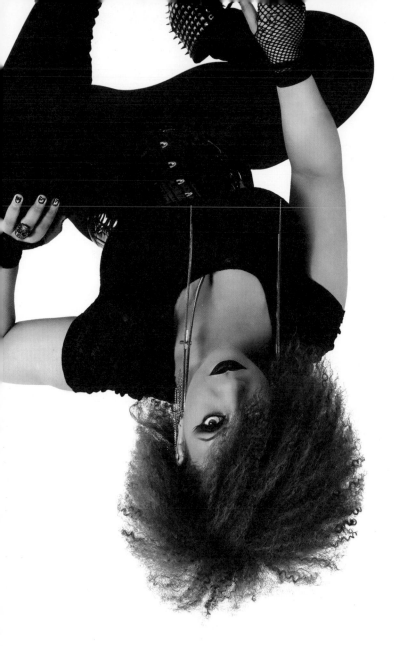

Hair colorist Mykey O'Halloran has seen a recent spike in green hair from its use in movies like *Suicide Squad*. Of course, for the Joker's hair, they used Manic Panic hair color! Mykey loves the variety of the shade: "First things first, before someone makes the leap to green hair, they would need to decide exactly what shade they'd like to achieve: A deep forest green, lizard green, slime green, flubber green, lime green, cactus green—there are many shades to choose from—as this decision would indicate how light they'd need to lift the hair first. The beauty about green is that you only need it to lift the hair to a golden hue because the deeper shades of green in the Manic Panic range, like Enchanted Forest and Green Envy, will counteract and cover any warmth that may persist after lifting.

ROCK 'N' ROLL GODDESS MILITIA VOX ROCKS GREEN ENVY HIGH VOLTAGE CLASSIC CREAM.
PHOTO BY YASSIR KETCHUM

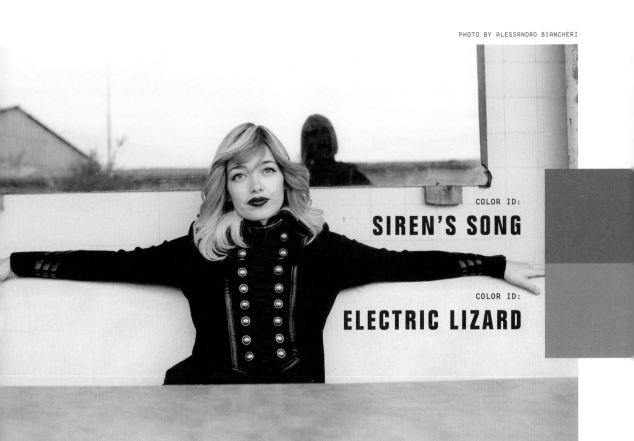

COLOR ID:

SIREN'S SONG

COLOR ID:

ELECTRIC LIZARD

"Any skin tone can pull off green hair, so it's more about deciding what level you would like the color to sit on. If someone is used to being brunette or having dark roots, my suggestion would be to do Enchanted Forest at the roots for a deep shade, and then melt it out into the brighter shades, like Green Envy or Electric Lizard. I personally like to do variations and shades of different greens throughout (example: Enchanted Forest, Venus Envy, and Green Envy) for a more earthy green shade at the root area, and then for the ends, a pastelized version of either or all three of those shades with a hint of Electric Lizard in some pieces throughout to make the colors really pop!

"You could even keep your natural dark roots and then melt them into green for a creative color ombré, a look directly influenced by the 1970s version of the Joker with his stretched, grown-out roots. I love the contrast of natural regrowth with green; it has a really punk feel to it—I can envision a punk with a green Mohawk that looks like a lizard's back, hairsprayed and set into place with natural brown regrowth and natural brown shaved sides—the contrast just makes the whole look work!"

THIS BEAUTIFUL STUDY IN CONTRASTING GREENS WAS CREATED BY OLIVIA IANNARELLI USING ELECTRIC LIZARD AND SIREN'S SONG.

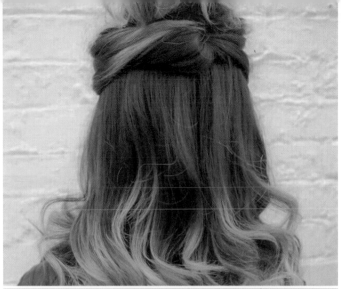

AUSTRALIAN STYLIST
ANGELA SKULLPTURES
CREATED THIS
BEAUTIFUL GREEN
COLOR MELT
USING ELECTRIC
BANANA AND
ENCHANTED FOREST.

PHOTO BY ANGELA SKULLPTURES

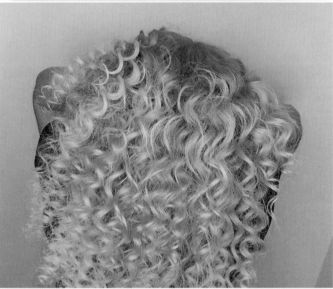

STYLISTS SAM
REECE AND DANIEL
BIGGIN CREATED
THIS BLUE TO NEON
GREEN COLOR MELT
USING MANIC PANIC
CLASSIC HIGH
VOLTAGE COLORS
ELECTRIC LIZARD,
ATOMIC TURQUOISE,
AND ELECTRIC
BANANA.

PHOTO BY SAM REECE & DANIEL BIGGIN

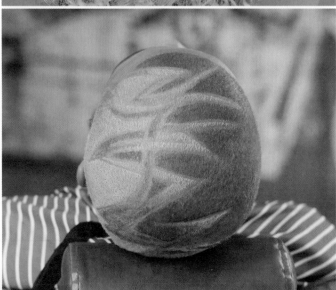

SHAROON TYLER'S
SIGNATURE
STYLE MIXES
GEOMETRY WITH
COLOROLOGY USING
ATOMIC TURQUOISE
AND ELECTRIC
LIZARD.

PHOTO BY SHAROON TYLER

COLOR OPTIONS FOR HAIR THAT IS NOT PRELIGHTENED (WE CALL IT A TOP COAT!)

Dye results on natural hair colors that are not prelightened will not be as intense and will typically wash out much faster. Some Manic Panic colors will provide a tint or glow of color that can be seen best in bright sunlight.

If your hair is naturally dark blond to dark brown, the following colors are good options if you don't want to prelighten:

SERPENTINE GREEN	GREEN ENVY	RAVEN
ENCHANTED FOREST	FUCHSIA SHOCK	PURPLE HAZE
CELESTINE BLUE	BLUE VELVET	DEEP PURPLE DREAM
VIOLET NIGHT	VAMPIRE RED	INFRA RED
ROCK 'N' ROLL RED	RED VELVET	HOT HOT PINK

Tish's favorite "top coat" is Fuchsia Shock. It's so strong and gives a beautiful maraschino cherry glow to most dark hair; plus it adds a glossy shine!

2. IF YOU REMEMBER THE '80s, YOU OBVIOUSLY WEREN'T THERE!

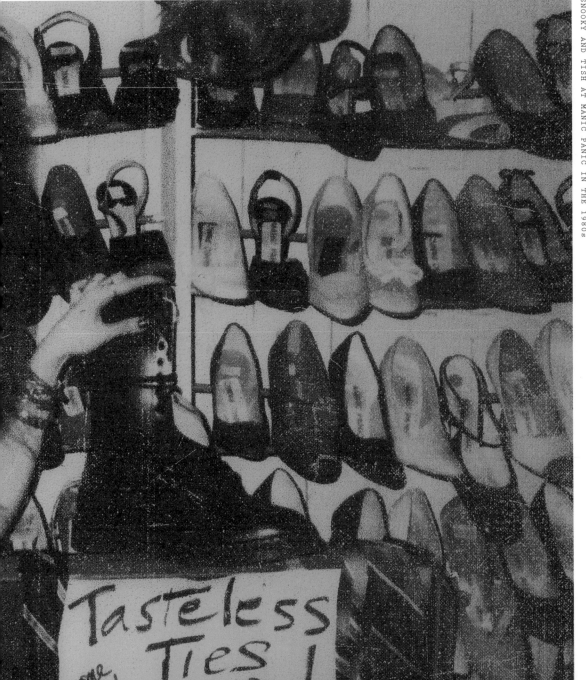

Tasteless Ties
some silk!
50¢

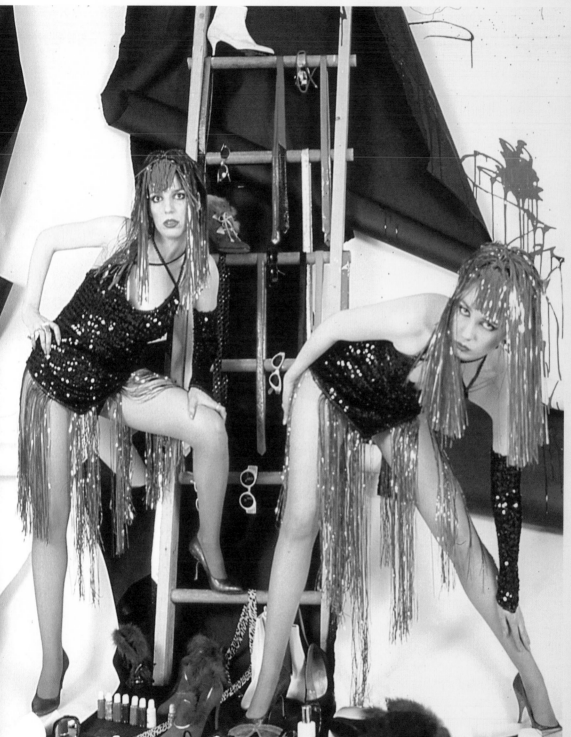

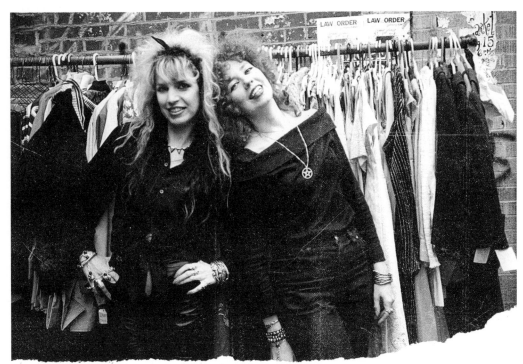

*T*ish and Snooky entered the 1980s with a bang! The Manic Panic storefront appeared in the opening credits of *Saturday Night Live*. This, along with the continued press coverage and good old-fashioned word of mouth, attracted an entirely new set of celebrity fans who ventured downtown to see what all the buzz was about. Everyone, including Meryl Streep, Paul Simon, Tony Curtis, Bill Murray, the Blues Brothers (John Belushi and Dan Aykroyd), Bruce Springsteen, Carrie Fisher, Caroline Kennedy, and Annie Lennox, frequented the shop during the '80s.

"I remember one day, it was the hottest day of the summer and we had no air conditioning. As I sat in the store all sweaty and miserable, I looked up and saw this fancy black car pull up. This woman dressed to the nines with big black curly hair in thigh-high boots and a miniskirt got out. I thought '*Ugh*, who is this chick from New Jersey going shopping dressed like that?!'" Snooky laughs. "I was just so hot and bothered, I didn't even get up to help her when she walked into the store. Then she spoke, and I realized it was Cher! I immediately jumped to attention and helped her find the makeup she wanted. I even sold her a Sic F*cks T-shirt and one of Tish's original designed dresses!" Tish jumps in with a giggle, "I may have already worn it once or twice at a gig...

"John Belushi was another big Manic Panic fan as well as being a fan of our band, the Sic F*cks. He said we had the 'best asses in NYC' and even introduced the band a few times, saying to the

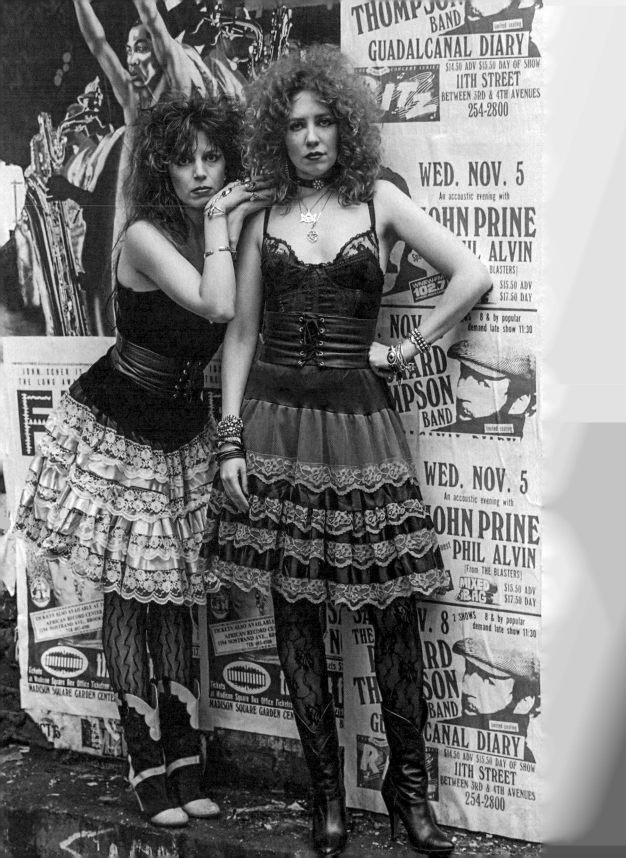

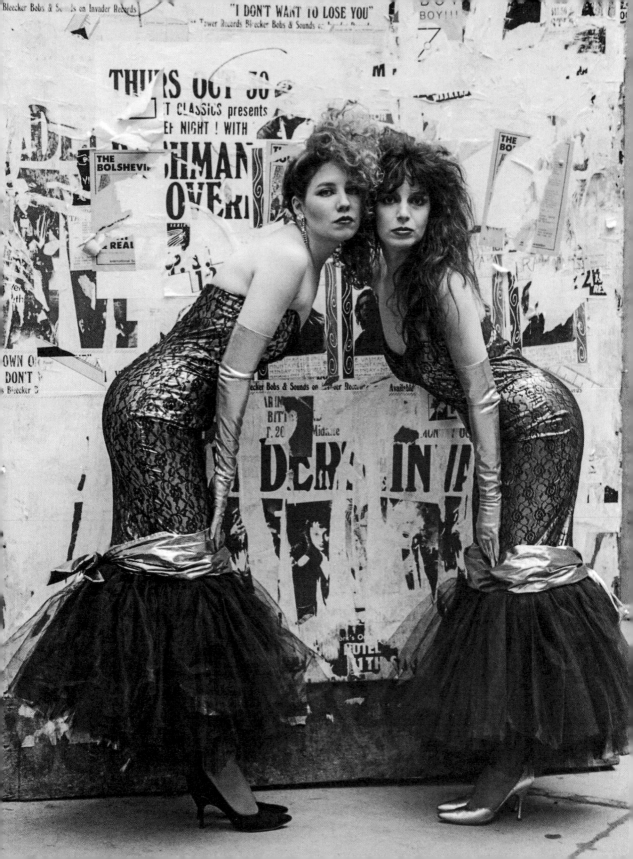

audience, 'Are ya hungry? Then EAT THIS! The Sic F*cks!'"

Tish remembers, "He'd drive up to the store in the Bluesmobile with Dan Aykroyd to buy our colored hairspray." They invited the girls to the last party they hosted at their Blues Club. It was Dan Aykroyd's birthday, and John asked them to do backup vocals for him and Dan. "I called my boyfriend to show off, bragging that I was going to do backup vocals for the Blues Brothers. He was like, 'So, who's the band playing?' I said, 'I don't know, some long-haired guys with big beards. They're called ZZ something or other?'" says Tish. "He screamed in the phone, 'ZZ Top?! Are you kidding?!' I was a punk rocker; I had no idea who they were!"

Musicians from all over the world were making their way to the doors of Manic Panic's storefront on St. Marks Place, the mecca for all things underground style. But the allure of their rapid business growth mixed with nationwide name recognition and press was attracting competitors, copycats, and those looking to make a quick buck off a trend. New retailers started to move into the area around St. Marks Place, some eventually becoming the neighbors from hell.

One of these direct competitors began adding punk fashion to his usual selection of vintage clothing. But how did he find it? He followed the girls overseas. "Every time we'd go over to England and bring back really cool stuff, like the Mary Quant socks, jumpsuits, tops, and pantyhose, our competitor down the block would send his employees in to see what we had in that was new," Snooky reminisces. "Then he'd fly over to England and get the same stuff we had. He then asked those vendors not to sell to us anymore! He said he could buy more and he wanted the exclusive."

Tish jumps in: "We got screwed out of many of the items we brought to market and made popular and almost everything

that we brought from London. But the only thing we didn't get screwed out of were beauty products. From there, we started specializing in cosmetics and beauty products. The male business owners down the street didn't know anything about the beauty market. We were not only punk women business owners but also actual singers/performers, so we knew what other women like us wanted.

"We had begun wholesaling hair color and cosmetics, and eventually started exhibiting at trade shows. Our products were well received at shows that catered to small, underground/alternative shops, but at the International Beauty Show, the stylists and beauty supply owners had no idea what to make of us. They were soooo NOT interested—they didn't have a clientele that wanted it. Most of the world had never seen hair colors like these, never mind know how to use them. Only some of the younger, more adventurous students were interested."

This decision to focus more on cosmetics and color in-store was crucial for Manic Panic's safety in the rocky financial and business climate. And in typical Tish and Snooky fashion, they made sure they got the last laugh. Tish says, "After our competitor went over to England and told everyone not to sell to us, we went back to one of the wholesale outlets in disguise and gave our cousin Jeanne's name and business information for her store in New Hampshire so that the warehouse manager at the outlet would let us shop." Snooky chimes in with a laugh: "But the entire time he'd be like, 'Don't I know you girls? You look kind of familiar!' Taking no for an answer is not in our vocabulary!"

But it wasn't just hair color and makeup that was dominating Manic Panic's sales during the '80s. The shop had become known as the go-to place to purchase wigs of all styles and colors, at-home bleach kits (which were nearly impossible to

The store was in many ways a community center. St. Marks was a central shopping location for locals and tourists. Friends, artists, and musicians would stop in on their way home from work, or while walking their dog. More often than not, people would come in to see Tish and Snooky, but we all became friends and acquaintances through this small shop if we hadn't already met at CBGB. Bands would stop in with their flyers or posters to hang up if they were playing that week. And no matter how odd or weird people seemed to be, Tish and Snooky would always welcome them into their circle. They were so accepting of other people.

THE EAST VILLAGE WAS FILLED WITH CHARACTERS.

It wasn't unusual to have a dominatrix come in with a client on a leash or couples who were dressed in rubber clothes. It was all part of the landscape back then and really seemed to be a place where people could be who they wanted to be, no matter how freaky that may have been at the time. One day I came in to work, and Alison East was behind the counter, standing on what appeared to be a rolled-up rug. I didn't realize that there was a PERSON rolled up in the rug. His name was Kevin, but we called him Floor. He was this normal-looking guy who liked to roll himself up in a rug and have people stand on him.

—ALISON AGUIAR

THANK GOODNESS YOU GUYS MAKE COLOR.... I'D BE LOST!

—CYNDI LAUPER

SHE'S SO UNUSUAL

While most female musicians during the 1980s were opting for big, teased-out hair, Cyndi Lauper topped them all with even wilder hair, with her own twist: By experimenting with Manic Panic shades of red, orange, and yellow, Lauper created what can only be described as a surreal sunset for the cover of her blockbuster 1983 debut album *She's So Unusual*. Lauper then dominated the MTV airwaves, bopping around her kitchen with wacky two-toned orange hues in "Girls Just Want to Have Fun" to singing sadly in bed with a half-shaved head and even more vivid orange locks in "Time After Time." Lauper proved early in her career that she was willing to take "shocking" beauty risks that no mainstream female artist had ever had the guts to do.

No wonder Lauper gravitated toward Tish and Snooky, becoming an early regular at the Manic Panic storefront. They first met at Irving Plaza in 1980 when their band Pin Ups played on the same bill as Cyndi's band Blue Angel, both opening for XTC. Snooky tells, "Cyndi has been a Manic Panic Dyehard since the 1980s, when she would shop in our store before she really made it big. Her growing popularity definitely aided in Manic Panic's success, giving us a lot more mainstream exposure all over the globe. For that we're eternally grateful." Tish chimes in: "And at the same time, Manic Panic hair color helped give Cyndi her iconic, colorful edge that most people at that time hadn't seen before, making her stand out amongst other artists and adding to her unusual, unconventional beauty!"

Still creating terrific music and coloring her hair with Manic Panic, Lauper recently rocked a gorgeous shade of Cotton Candy Pink. She told fashion and beauty website Fashion Unfiltered, "If I get a little down or am just plain tired, I go color my hair, put some lipstick on, and feel good again."

find during this period in time), and hair color spray.

Tish recalls, "We sold a ton of colored hairspray at the time—it was the '80s; big hair was in!" Snooky jumps in: "Back then, we used to buy the colored hairspray we sold from a Halloween and party supply company. They were totally shocked because we were buying it all year round!"

Tish laughs. "We were buying so much but our store was so tiny. Boxes of hairspray were piled sky-high, jammed behind the clothing racks. One time around Halloween, one of our employees got to the store to find that an entire pallet of the hair color spray had been delivered. They just left it outside. She was so pissed because she had to bring the boxes in one by one, all by herself."

At the height of the store's fame, St. Marks Place was rapidly becoming more gentrified and marketed as a downtown shopping destination by Realtors. Since the media had extensively covered the success of the punk rock store, more and more retailers were moving in near St. Marks. And it wasn't just small shops. "When the Gap moved in, that was the beginning of the end," Tish reflects sadly. "There was no more room for small businesses because spaces got taken up by bigger, more generic clothing companies."

Tish continues: "Because of Manic Panic getting such publicity and notoriety, the neighborhood was getting 'hot.' We had asked the original landlord if we could buy the building from him, but he kept saying no. All of a sudden,

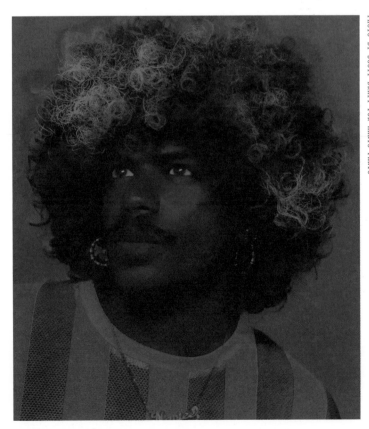

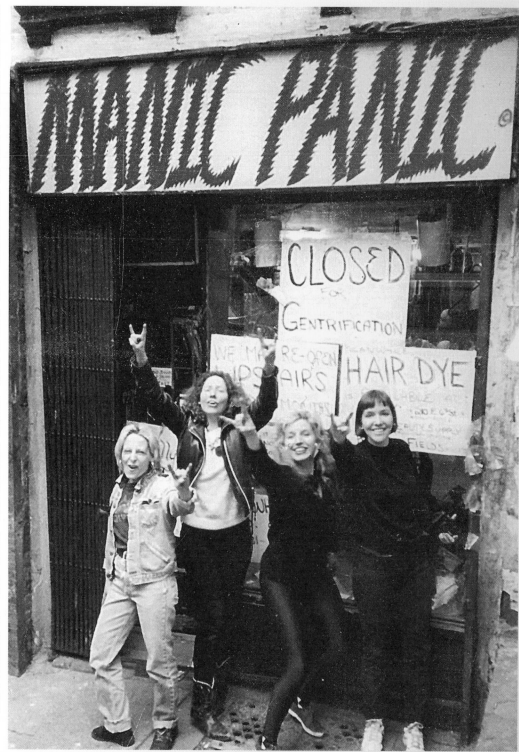

MANIC PANIC BOUTIQUE CLOSING FOR GENTRIFICATION, 1989 (LEFT TO RIGHT: SUZANNE REINHARDT-KUHN, SNOOKY, TISH, AND MARGARET McKAY)

THERE IS NOTHING MORE RARE, NOR MORE BEAUTIFUL, THAN A WOMAN BEING UNAPOLOGETICALLY HERSELF; COMFORTABLE IN HER PERFECT IMPERFECTION. TO ME, THAT IS THE TRUE ESSENCE OF BEAUTY.

—STEVE MARABOLI

around 1987, the building was sold. Our new landlord came in and said, 'I'm not renewing your lease.' We talked to him and told him, 'We're the reason your building is worth anything at all! We pioneered the neighborhood and now you're throwing us out?!' After that, he felt bad and let us stay month to month for a while, but then gave us two weeks' notice."

The girls suggested he let them rent the space upstairs, which was an apartment at the time but could be made into a store, as it would be less expensive. He loved the idea and told them once the renovations were completed in about three months that they could move back in. "We put everything in storage," says Snooky, "and started doing wholesale orders out of my boyfriend Andy's tiny, walk-up studio apartment. He'd come home to us in there answering the phone, taking orders, packing orders—we had giant boxes of hair dye piled up to the ceiling! At the time, he was probably ready to murder me, but we got married instead.

"In addition to losing our store, we lost our weekend gig at Sophie's Honky Tonk on Avenue A. Eddy Dixon and the Dixonettes had played there for years, until Sophie, a woman in her eighties, was forced out by gentrification."

"We were just doing everything ourselves," Tish says, chiming back in. "Snooky had an old station wagon, so we'd throw the boxes to be shipped into the car. Snooky would drive like crazy to UPS while I was still packing orders in the back seat." Three months of renovation on the store turned into an entire year. "When our landlord was finally finished renovating, he said to us, 'Actually, I changed my mind. The rent is going to be much higher than we had discussed before.' So we looked at each other and said, 'Screw it,' and continued to work out of the apartment for a while."

When the Manic Panic storefront officially closed its doors in 1989, it was the end of an era for authentic punk rockers in St. Marks Place. But this setback didn't stop Tish and Snooky from trying to find another spot in the neighborhood they had helped popularize.

Snooky was at a party talking to Doug Levine, who owned Crunch Fitness. He told her he had a part of his Crunch space in a basement on St. Marks Place that he wasn't using. So they rented out his little basement, which was—literally and figuratively—a step down. But something good always comes out of hardship, and the sisters learned a

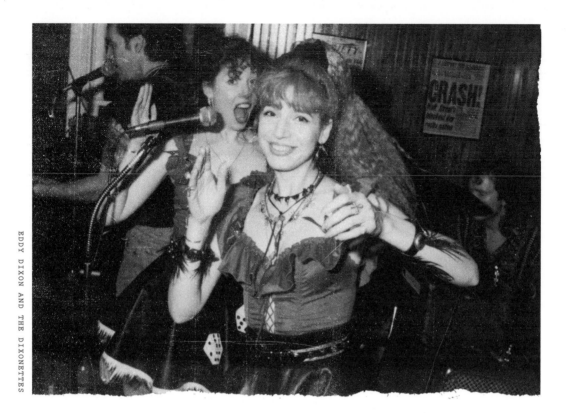

lot about business just by being next door to Doug. "He taught us how to negotiate rates with credit card companies and to always blame your accountant for EVERYTHING," says Tish, laughing. "He was probably the first bona fide business owner we knew. We'd play a game with him called 'Who's cheaper?' and would recount our latest acts of frugality, competing with each other to see who was cheaper. Doug would always win the game!"

"People didn't want to go downstairs to our new location because it was a little scary," says Snooky, "but we were only there for a short while. When his lease was up, ours was, too, so once again we had nowhere to go. We weren't very good at planning ahead."

The moving truck was coming to take all of the Manic Panic stock to storage when good luck struck again. A landlord who had shown the girls a space on East Ninth Street happened to stop by, asking if they were still interested. "We were like, 'Yeah, we'd love to take it!' and he was like, 'Great! When would you like to move in?' And we said, 'Uh...now?'" Tish laughs. "It was perfect timing! So instead of bringing everything to storage like we had planned, we brought it straight over to our new space. He was so cool. He said, 'Okay, I'll go get a lease and we can sign it later. Here's the key!'"

At the end of the 1980s, Tish and Snooky had found themselves kicked out of their beloved original store and were trying to build their business without a permanent home for Manic Panic. While things may have seemed like they were taking a turn for the worse, in reality, the girls were about to embark on an entirely new venture in the 1990s: manufacturing.

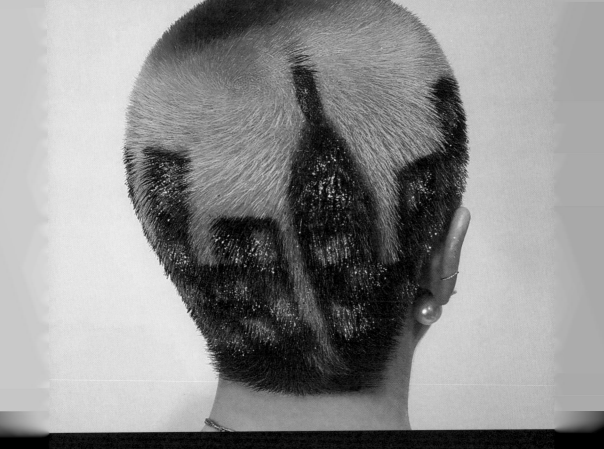

WHEN TO DIY VS. WHEN YOU NEED PROFESSIONAL HELP

When deciding whether to DIY with your Manic Panic hair color at home or go see a professional hair colorist, first consider your expertise. Is this the first time you are coloring your hair? Has your hair been processed a lot? Is your hair currently colored? If so, see a professional hair colorist.

Regardless of your hair color experience, if you need to get a complicated process or any type of advanced bleach job, it's always recommended to see a professional hair colorist. Bleaching an entire

However, once you've seen a professional hair colorist to do the initial double process and color, you may be able to continue bleaching at home for any root touch-ups by using the Manic Panic Flash Lightning Bleach Kits if you feel comfortable enough with this method. But as stated earlier, NEVER EVER overlap the bleach over previously bleached hair. If you're someone who likes the grown-out-roots look, you can continue to simply color the rest of your hair at home using Manic

YELLOW HAIR!

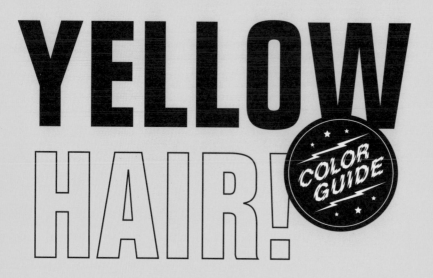

COLOR GUIDE

IT'S ELECTRIC [BANANA],
SO FRIGHTFULLY HECTIC!

MANIC PANIC CLASSIC HIGH VOLTAGE AND PROFESSIONAL COLORS

ELECTRIC BANANA	SUNSHINE	SOLAR YELLOW

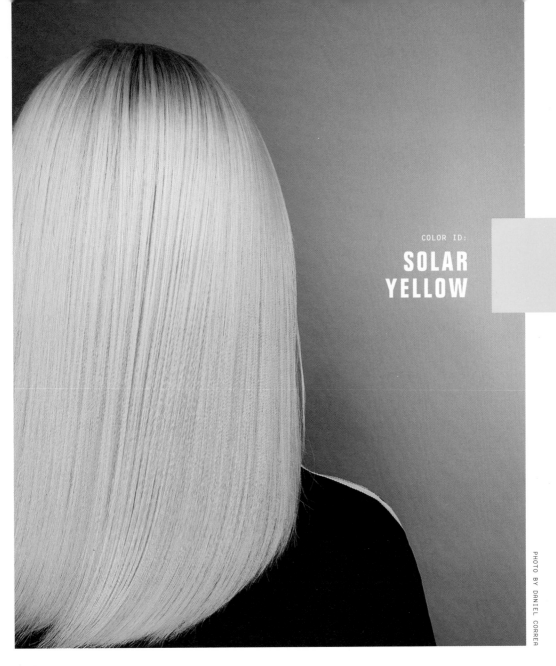

PHOTO BY DANIEL CORREA

MANIC PANIC CHILEAN STYLIST DANIEL CORREA TAKES US FROM PLATINUM TO YELLOW USING SOLAR YELLOW.

t's not often you associate a person with a color, but for hair colorist and literal ray of light Mischa G., she is the embodiment of all things yellow: "After being a bleach blonde for years, it made the most sense for me to switch over to yellow since it's one of the easiest hair colors to maintain, and it also made me feel like a cartoon character," she tells.

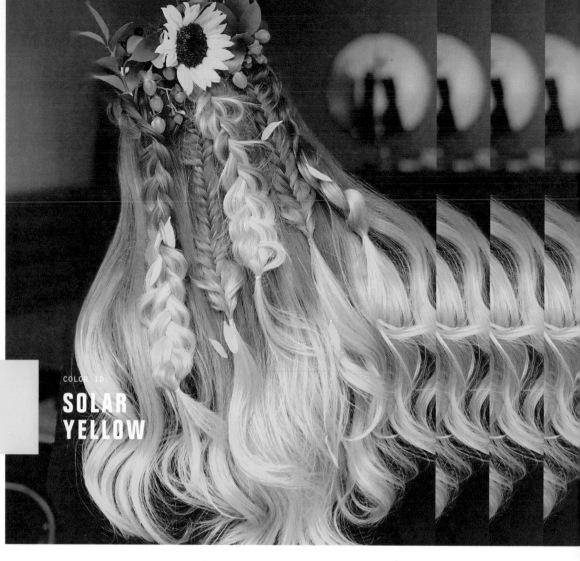

COLOR ID:
SOLAR YELLOW

BRAND AMBASSADOR CHELSEA MANFRE CREATED THIS BEAUTIFUL FLORAL FANTASY USING SMOKESCREEN, DIVINE WINE, RED VELVET, SOLAR YELLOW, CELESTINE BLUE, AND SERPENTINE GREEN.

For the last eight years, Mischa's been sporting nothing but yellow locks, becoming known in the New York City hair circuit as the infamous yellow-haired stylist. But yellow wouldn't be such a popular hair color nowadays without certain pop culture icons—such as Cyndi Lauper, Divine, and Amanda Lepore—leading the way first.

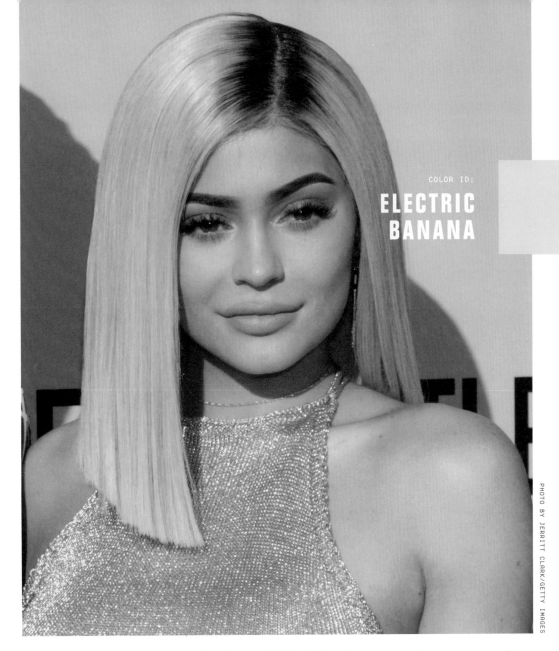

COLOR ID:

ELECTRIC BANANA

KYLIE JENNER TAKES YELLOW TO SOARING NEW HEIGHTS WITH THIS DAY-GLO MIXTURE OF ELECTRIC BANANA AND ELECTRIC LIZARD.

Here, the queen of yellow dishes on how you can create your very own sunshine in a bottle at home. "I wish more people would embrace yellow hair! It was such a popular color in the punk movement because it was anti-blond, anti-beach blond, anti–Barbie blond. It was the, 'Hey, my hair is yellow! Crayon yellow! Deal with it, blondie.' My favorite yellow hair moment of all time was when Amanda Lepore was rocking it in her iconic video with MAC Cosmetics®, where she's rubbing pink lipstick all over her lips and face. That was so punk rock.

THE BEAUTIFUL IS ALWAYS BIZARRE.

—CHARLES BAUDELAIRE

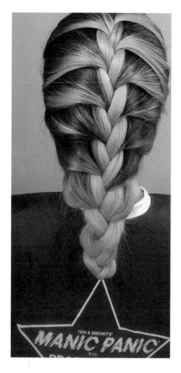

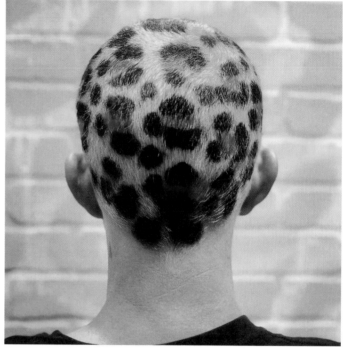

ABOVE LEFT
STYLIST LAURA CHIVU MAKES
YELLOW HAIR WEARABLE WITH THIS
SOFT BRAID COLORED WITH SOLAR
YELLOW AND LOVE POWER PURPLE.

PHOTO BY LAURA CHIVU

ABOVE RIGHT
AYUMI MITSUISHI IS KNOWN FOR
HER HAND-PAINTED LEOPARD-PRINT
HAIR. SHE GIVES "TRADITIONAL"
LEOPARD-PRINT HAIR AN ADDED POP
BY USING A YELLOW BASE LIKE
ELECTRIC BANANA ACCENTED WITH
ELECTRIC LAVA AND RAVEN.

PHOTO BY AYUMI MITSUISHI

"The great thing about yellow hair dye is that you can transition right to it from your current shade of blond. You don't have to get your hair to be white blond before making it yellow; you can just bleach it for about fifteen to twenty minutes instead and go straight from there.

"I personally like to use Manic Panic's Sunshine and mix in a few drops of Psychedelic Sunset, which is an orange, to give it that perfect macaroni-and-cheese yellow color. I prefer using Sunshine on myself because most of my color scheme in what I wear is kind of that '70s yellow, grandma's couch tone. If you want something more vibrant and neon, go straight for Electric Banana, or you can even mix it with Sunshine and experiment with your own shade of yellow.

"Another great thing about yellow hair dye is that you can touch up hair right in the shower. Just comb the yellow hair dye through, leave it on for the duration of your shower, and then rinse it out. If you do this in-shower method, the dye itself won't discolor your hands or anything. However, if you're using it on dry hair, I recommend wearing gloves just for safety. Either way, you can touch up yellow by yourself every two weeks or so—it's probably the easiest color you can maintain yourself at home."

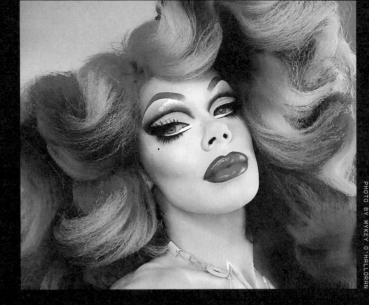

PHOTO BY MYKEY O'HALLORAN

DRAG QUEENS RULE

Long before *RuPaul's Drag Race* became a pop culture phenomenon, drag performers were perfecting the art form in NYC downtown clubs. Tish recalls, "We were 'hags' from the time we hit our teens. We were fascinated not only by the queens but also by gay bars and drag clubs themselves, with the amazing music you wouldn't hear anywhere else, and the lip-synched drag shows you wouldn't see anywhere else."

Their earliest interactions with groundbreaking drag performers were formative, to say the least. They watched in awe as Dom DeLuise, in full drag, judged a Halloween costume contest at one of the popular clubs.

"In the basement dressing room of the Palm Casino Revue, we learned almost everything we needed to know about hair, wigs, and stage makeup from our drag queen friends and fellow performers. Gorilla Rose would 'modernize' tired old wigs from the 1960s by putting them on backward. The nape of the neck became the bangs, and the rest of the hair would fall into sort of a shag, that could be back-combed into a whole new look. We learned the art of layering sets of ultrathick false lashes—one pair was never enough!—covering brows with eyebrow putty/wax topped with thick foundation, then drawing on new ones above, and contouring to create the illusion of cheekbones on a chubby face and even large breasts on a flat chest—that certainly came in handy!" says Snooky, laughing.

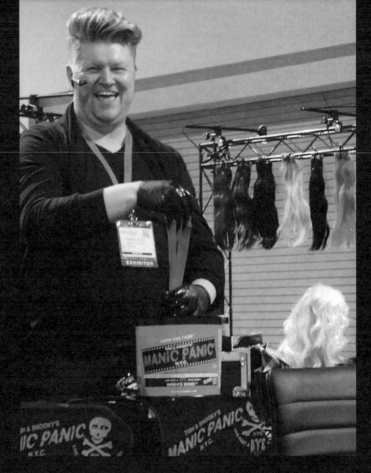

CHECK OUT THIS STEP-BY-STEP
CREATION OF A BEAUTIFUL WIG BY
RENOWNED STYLIST DANIEL KOYE
USING DIVINE WINE, LOVE POWER
PURPLE, AND PUSSYCAT PINK.

DIP DYEING
WITH DANIEL KOYE

The best way to dye your wigs and extensions is by dip dyeing. It
will give an all-over saturation of the hair and you can see the final
results, so you will be able to amp up the color or tweak it. Here's
how Daniel dip-dyes his wigs and extensions.

1. BRUSH THE HAIR AND SMOOTH IT ALL IN THE SAME DIRECTION.

2. GET A COLOR-SAFE BOWL OR TUB THAT CAN HOLD A GALLON OF WATER OR MORE.

3. FORMULATE YOUR COLOR. MIX YOUR COLOR IN A COLOR BOWL AND TEST IT BY DOING A STRAND TEST. THIS STEP WILL HELP ACHIEVE THE DESIRED COLOR FOR YOUR WIG. ONCE YOU FIGURE OUT YOUR FORMULA, YOU WILL WANT ABOUT 4 OUNCES OF COLOR TO HALF GALLON OF WATER.

Tip: If your wig needs a refresher, you can use half of the product from step #4 and do a quick dunk to revive the color.

4. FILL YOUR COLOR-SAFE TUB OR BOWL WITH A HALF GALLON OF THE HOTTEST WATER YOU CAN HANDLE, BEING EXTRA CAREFUL NOT TO MAKE IT TOO HOT.

5. TAKE YOUR FINAL COLOR MIX AND DUMP IT INTO THE HOT WATER.

6. MIX UNTIL THE COLOR IS DISSOLVED COMPLETELY. WE RECOMMEND USING A SPOON SO YOU DON'T BURN YOUR HANDS.

7. NOW DIP THE HAIR INTO YOUR MIXTURE AS EVENLY AS POSSIBLE FOR THE FIRST DUNK. THIS WILL HELP THE HAIR ABSORB THE COLOR EVENLY.

8. DUNK SEVERAL TIMES AND CHECK THE COLOR. USE A CLIP OR A HANGER AND PIN THE WIG OR EXTENSION FOR DUNKING.

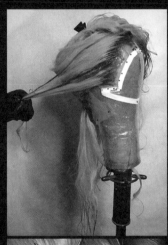

9. FOR AN INTENSE COLOR, LEAVE THE HAIR IN THE COLOR FOR 30 MINUTES OR MORE. THE LONGER YOU KEEP IT IN, THE MORE THE COLOR WILL ABSORB. WHEN YOU TAKE OUT THE HAIR, THE LEFTOVER WATER WILL COME OUT CLEAR, AS THE HAIR HAS SOAKED UP ALL THE COLOR. IF THERE IS NO COLOR LEFT IN THE WATER AND YOU WANT A RICHER LOOK, YOU CAN DO ANOTHER DIP-DYE PROCESS.

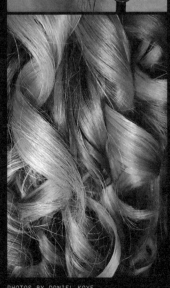

10. RINSE WITH COLD WATER. THIS IS IMPORTANT TO LOCK IN THAT COLOR.

11. LET THE HAIR DRIP DRY. THIS WILL HELP THE CUTICLE CLOSE.

12. BLOCK YOUR WIG OR EXTENSIONS AND STYLE AS DESIRED.

PHOTOS BY DANIEL KOYE

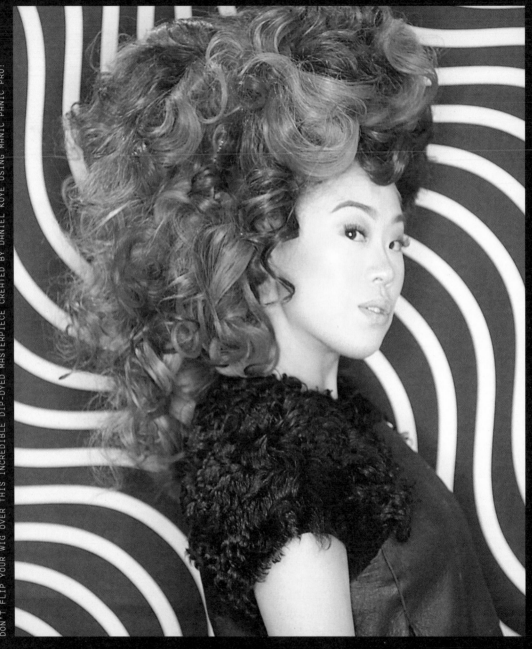

BEAUTY BEGINS THE MOMENT
YOU DECIDE TO BE YOURSELF.

—COCO CHANEL

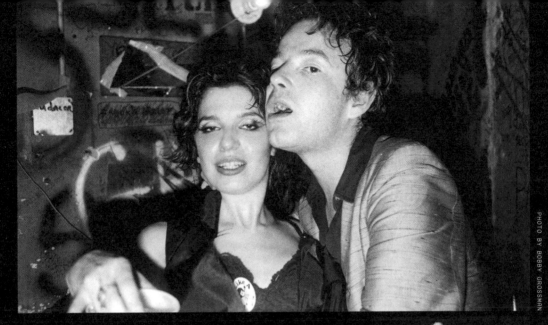

TISH AND WARHOL SUPERSTAR JACKIE CURTIS

The original Manic Panic boutique on St. Marks Place was a haven for those who marched to the beat of a different drum, so drag queens were no strangers to the store. Queens who performed at the nearby Club 57 and Pyramid Club—such as Ethyl Eichelberger, Hapi Phace, Hattie Hathaway, Lypsinka, Lady Bunny, and all the "Boy Bar Beauties" from right down the block—would buy their wigs, lashes, and makeup at Manic Panic for a special discounted price. "We also performed there quite a bit, one time in drag as 'the Infamous Creamatelli Brothers,'" says Tish. "We may still hold the title of 'the world's creepiest drag kings.'"

The sisters love watching the career rise of RuPaul. He started out as a friend and customer in NYC in the late 1980s and hired Tish and Snooky to sing backup on his first album, *Star Booty*, as well as at a live performance at the Saint. You can see all three featured in the B-52's video "Good Stuff" dancing in a sea of bubbles. They're thrilled that he has evolved into such an inspirational role model and trailblazer in the community, not to mention an Emmy-winning entertainer! When he launched RuPaul's DragCon in 2015, Manic Panic was destined to be part of it. "We're so proud that we've been exhibiting at DragCon since its inception," says Tish. "And we're thrilled that it's getting bigger every year."

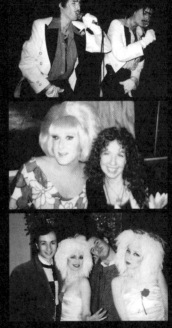

TOP
TISH AND SNOOKY AS THE INFAMOUS CREAMATELLI BROTHERS AT BOY BAR IN THE LATE '80s

MIDDLE
WIG-WEARING DRAG GODDESS, THE ONE AND ONLY LADY BUNNY, WITH SNOOKY, AS SHOT BY MICHAEL LOUIS

BOTTOM
FILMMAKER FENTON BAILEY, TISH, FILMMAKER RANDY BARBATO, AND SNOOKY AT LIMELIGHT

TO ME, BEAUTY IS ABOUT BEING COMFORTABLE IN YOUR OWN SKIN. IT'S ABOUT KNOWING AND ACCEPTING WHO YOU ARE.

—ELLEN DeGENERES

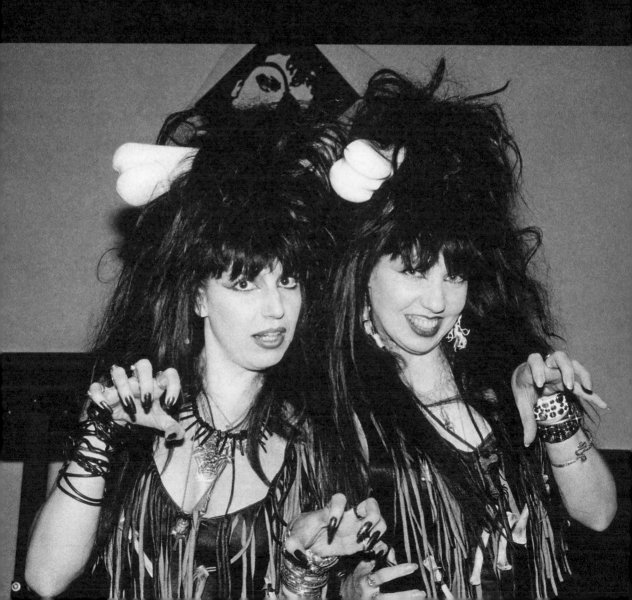

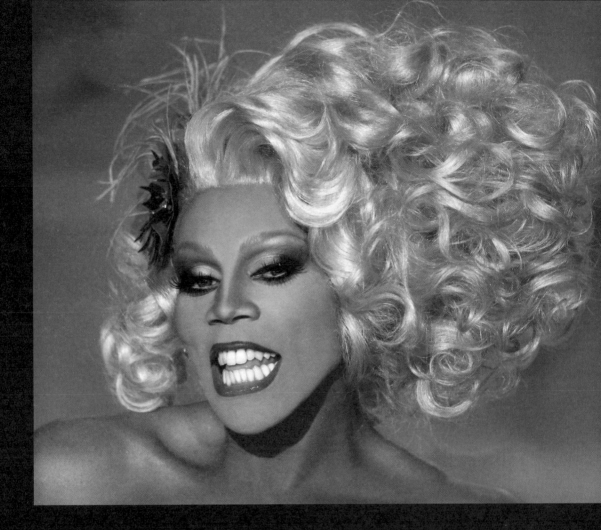

ABOVE
GO FOR THE GOLD WITH *DRAG RACE*
HOST RUPAUL IN THIS YELLOW-
TONED BLOND WIG.

PHOTO BY MARK BOSTER/GETTY IMAGES

RIGHT
SNOOKY AND TISH WITH THE
ONE AND ONLY RUPAUL AT THE
FIRST RUPAUL'S DRAGCON IN
LOS ANGELES, 2015

OPPOSITE
TISH AND SNOOKY AT CLUB 57

PHOTO BY ANDE WHYLAND

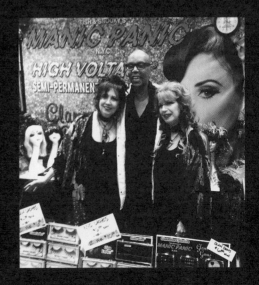

ORANGE

YOU GLAD YOU DYED YOUR HAIR?

COLOR GUIDE

MANIC PANIC CLASSIC HIGH VOLTAGE AND AMPLIFIED COLORS

ELECTRIC TIGER LILY

PSYCHEDELIC SUNSET

CORALLINE DREAM

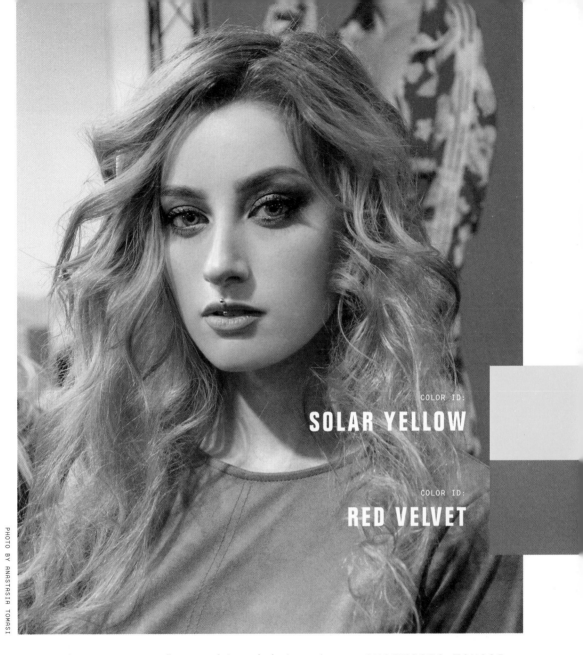

COLOR ID:
SOLAR YELLOW

COLOR ID:
RED VELVET

O n the same spectrum as yellow, orange hair was also having a major moment in the 1980s. Everyone from David Bowie, Kate Pierson of the B-52's, and the popular Troll Dolls had their heads ablaze in hues of orange. Hair colorist Roxie Darling tells how you, too, can achieve a perfect head of sunset (or tequila sunrise!) tones.

ANASTASIA TOMASI CREATED THIS FIERY REDHEAD USING MANIC PANIC PROFESSIONAL AT COSMOPROF BOLOGNA 2018.

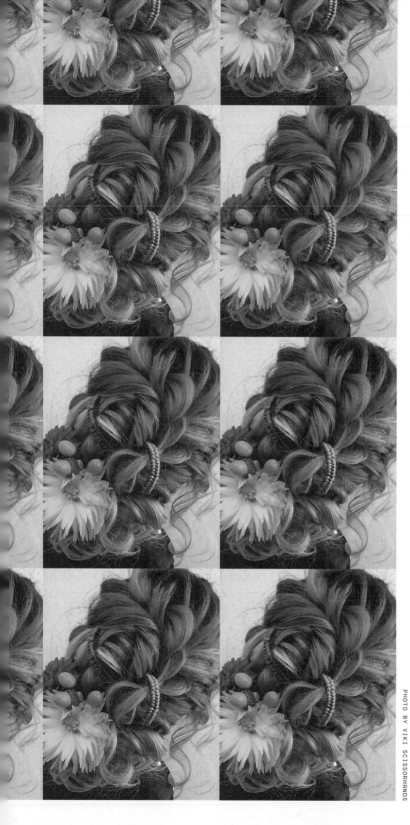

VIKI SCISSORHANDS
CREATED THIS
BEAUTIFUL AUTUMNAL
RED BOUQUET USING
MANIC PANIC PRO
RED VELVET,
SOLAR YELLOW,
PUSSYCAT PINK,
LOVE POWER PURPLE,
SMOKESCREEN, AND
PASTEL-IZER.

PHOTO BY VIKI SCISSORHANDS

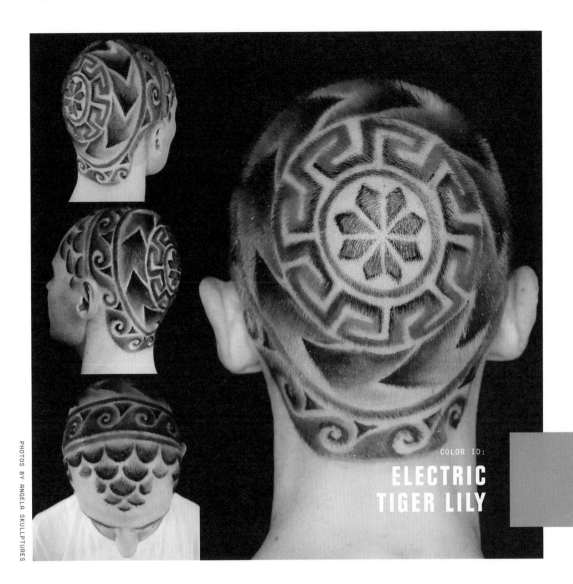

COLOR ID:

ELECTRIC TIGER LILY

"There is also something so sexual and abundant about the color orange. I think orange is hot and intense, and an artist like David Bowie was bringing those exact emotions out through his work, expressing himself with fearless abandon. He was very aware of how sexual he was. Ultimately, he did all of us a great service by being himself because it allowed everyone, despite their gender, permission to do the same.

"Orange hair is really punk because it is so unconventional. Although orange is typically a happy color, it's also a color that makes some people uncomfortable. Orange triggers our fight-or-flight response in the body, so it can also be abrasive in the way that it makes people feel, which is punk at its very core.

ANGELA SKULLPTURES CREATED THIS AMAZING HAIR MANDALA USING SUNSHINE, ELECTRIC TIGER LILY, PILLARBOX RED, AND RAVEN.

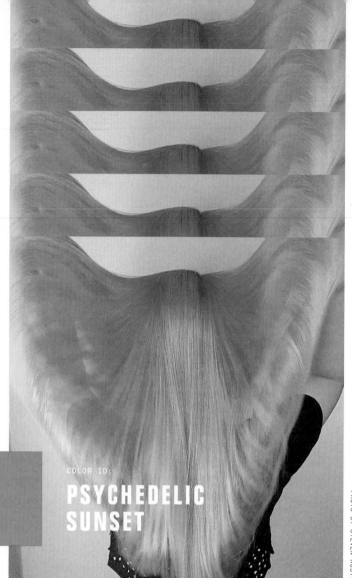

PHOTO BY STEVEN AUSTIN

COLOR ID:

PSYCHEDELIC SUNSET

STEVEN AUSTIN COMPLETELY BLEW US AWAY WITH THIS FLOWING MANE OF ELECTRIC BANANA, PSYCHEDELIC SUNSET, AND HOT HOT PINK.

"The process of going orange is very similar to going red, but it depends on if you want a peachy-orange or a red-orange. If you want something peachier, you'll want to bleach the hair using 20 volume and lifting to a medium yellow; this way it can have more light passing through it. If you want a red-orange, you only need to bleach the hair for a little bit, because there is so much natural orange in the hair and you'll want to retain that to have a really voluptuous red-orange.

"For a more red-orange, my favorite combination of Manic Panic's colors is mixing Electric Sunshine together with Vampire Red. For a peachy-orange, I love to mix Psychedelic Sunset with a few drops of Hot Hot Pink and Electric Lava."

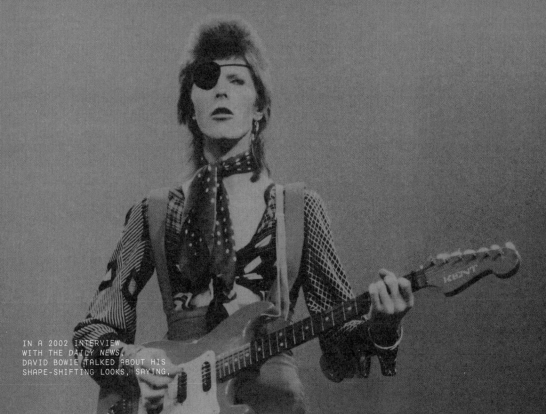

IN A 2002 INTERVIEW
WITH THE *DAILY NEWS*,
DAVID BOWIE TALKED ABOUT HIS
SHAPE-SHIFTING LOOKS, SAYING,

"Glam really did plant seeds for a new identity. I think a lot of kids needed that sense of

REINVENTION.

Kids learned that however crazy you may think it is, there is a place for what you want to do and who you want to be. And I needed that myself. Even though I was very shy, I found I could get onstage if I had a new identity."

PHOTO BY
GIJSBERT HANEKROOT/GETTY IMAGES

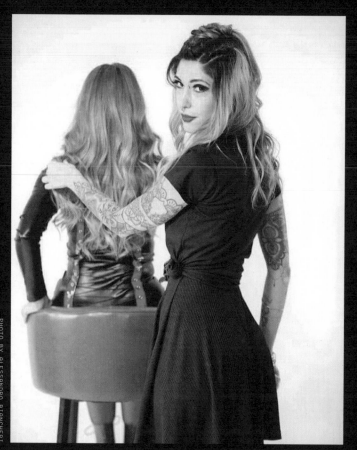

ANASTASIA TOMASI CREATED THIS BEAUTIFUL RAINBOW USING MANIC PANIC PROFESSIONAL DURING OUR 2018 EU TOUR.

PHOTO BY ALESSANDRO BIANCHERI

FINDING THE RIGHT HAIR COLORIST

While Manic Panic is all about DIY moxie, it's always great to get your hair colored by a pro! Finding the right hair colorist may often feel challenging or intimidating to a beginner, but don't let it keep you from following your rainbow-colored dreams! Whether you live in a big city or a smaller suburban area, the best thing you can do first is *research, research, research*. Check local review sites like Yelp, or if you see someone's hair color you like, ask them, "Who does your hair?" Trust us, they will be flattered.

Either way, once you track down a potential salon, go to its website and browse through the hair colorists' portfolios to see if any of them are a match for what you're looking for. Once you get the hair colorist's name, you can also check out their social media platforms—like Instagram, Facebook, or personal website—to get a better sense of their past work and experience working with creative color.

After you find someone you like, call or email the salon directly to set up a hair color consultation with the hair colorist. Make sure you come prepared with reference photos of the hair color you want, as well as any questions or concerns you may have about the process. It's helpful to jot down notes beforehand. During this hair color consultation, see if the salon carries Manic Panic. If they do, request the color you want to ensure they have it in stock on the day of your appointment. If they don't, tell them you'll bring it yourself. Don't accept imitations.

On that day, you'll want to prepare yourself to sit for anywhere between two and ten hours, depending on the complexity of your color. Make sure you come equipped with a cell phone charger; easy-to-eat, non-messy snacks; a book and/or magazine; and anything else that can keep you entertained. Most importantly, make sure you wear something comfortable.

Try to stay calm during the process. If this is your first time getting your hair bleached, be warned your hair may turn yellow or orange first and that your scalp might tingle slightly. This is all perfectly normal, and your hair colorist will likely apply a gentle hair treatment post-bleach to comfort and soothe your scalp. Unless your hair colorist appears to be doing something radically different than what you discussed or if you're in any kind of distress, trust them to be the professional artist they are.

Once you're all finished with your hair color (and done staring at your luscious new colored locks in the mirror), make sure to tip your hair colorist. If you really love your new look, tag them in any social media photos you post of your new hair color, so they can add to their portfolio. This will help someone else who's in the same situation as you were when you started. Be sure to ask your colorist when they recommend you come back for either a root touch-up, a new all-over hair dye color, or both.

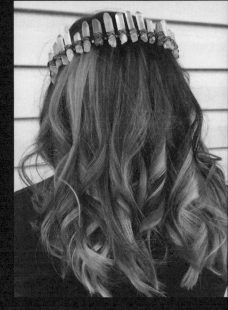

QUARTZ CRYSTALS WERE THE INSPIRATION FOR THIS STYLISH MIX USING MANIC PANIC PROFESSIONAL BY STYLIST OLIVIA FINAMORE.

PHOTO BY OLIVIA FINAMORE

3

RIOT BUSINESS GRRRLS IN THE 1990s:

TURNING HEADS AND TURNING WILD HAIR COLOR INTO A BRAND

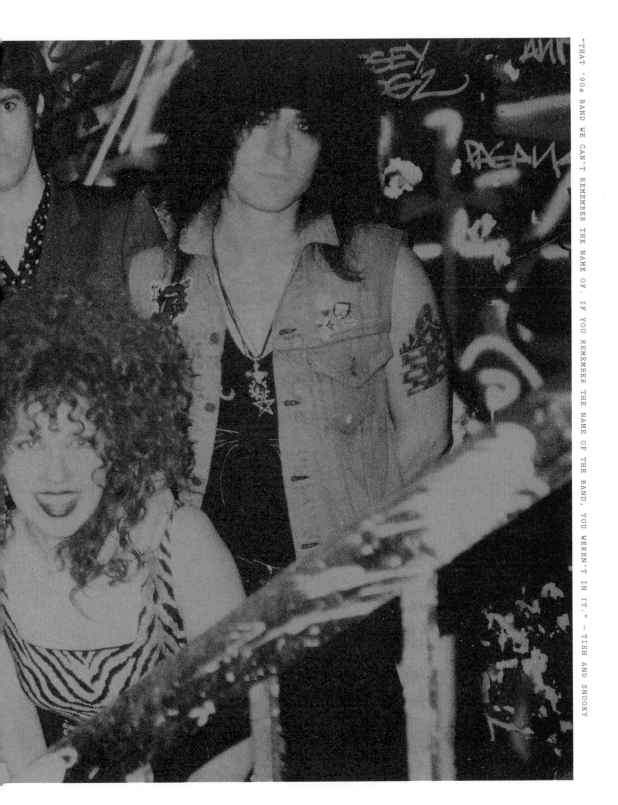

"THAT '90s BAND WE CAN'T REMEMBER THE NAME OF. IF YOU REMEMBER THE NAME OF THE BAND, YOU WEREN'T IN IT." — TISH AND SNOOKY

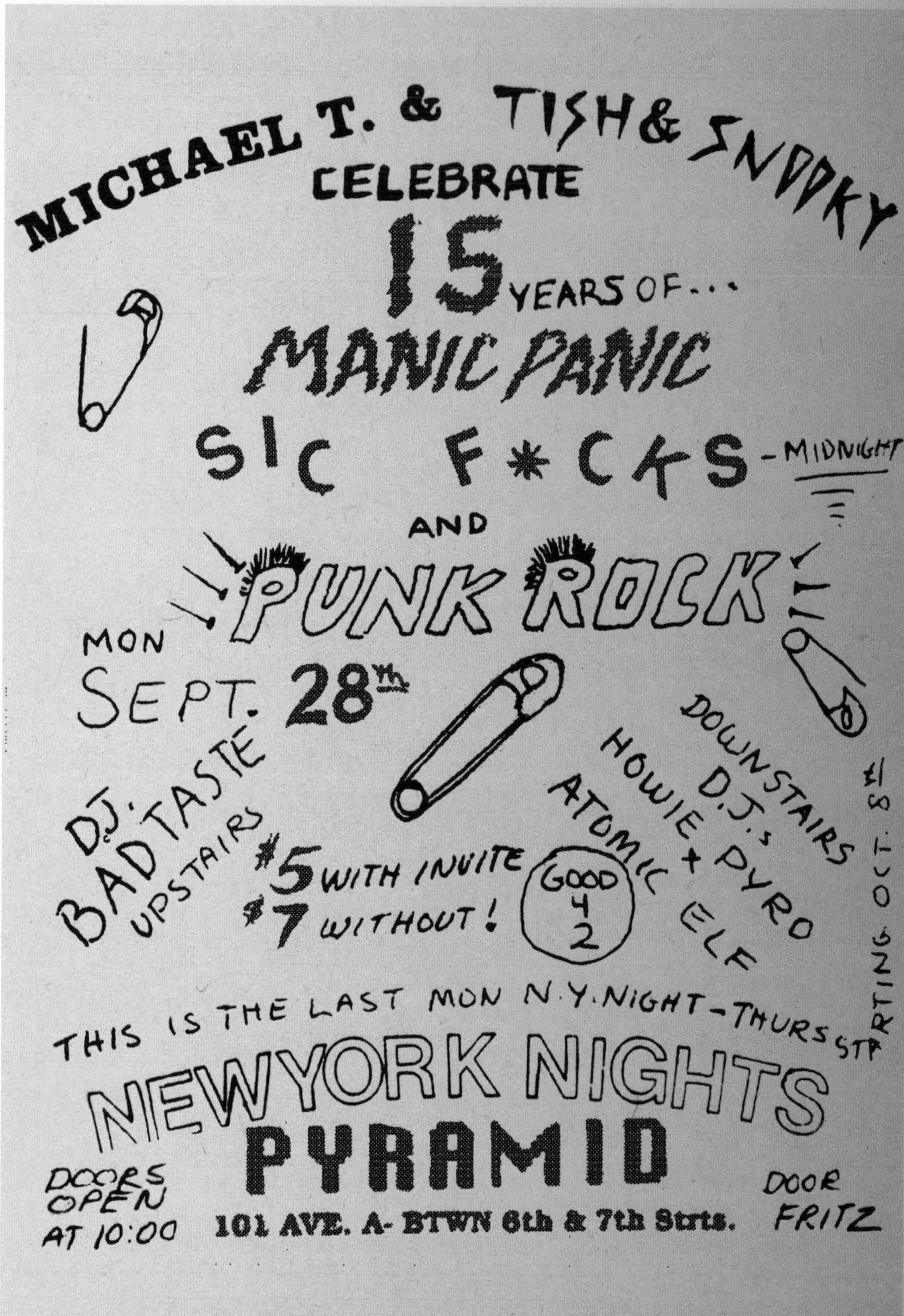

MANIC PANIC'S FIFTEEN YEAR MANNIVERSARY AT PYRAMID

As the 1990s began, East Coast punk and glam were slowly being replaced by West Coast grunge, alternative rock, and riot grrrl bands, mostly hailing from cities like Olympia, Seattle, and Los Angeles. While touring the country, these groups brought their own set of hair trends along with them. Unbrushed and unkempt, members of bands such as Nirvana, Hole, Bikini Kill, the Smashing Pumpkins, No Doubt, Babes in Toyland, L7, Red Hot Chili Peppers, the Murmurs, Lunachicks, and Green Day sported Manic Panic-colored hair, styles that teenagers around the country tried to emulate at home in their bathroom sinks.

While everyone else was grunge and serious, Tish and Snooky continued with the Sic F*cks while also going retro/glam/comedy lounge.

"We were in an act called Rocco Primavera and His New Jersey Nightingales," says Snooky. "It was a tongue-in-cheek lounge act. Fred Rothbell-Mista, who was one of the head honchos at the Limelight, a beautiful church turned nightclub, played Rocco. He wore a huge red pompadour wig, flashy outdated tuxedoes with gold chains. We played his gum-chewing, dumb blond sidekicks, wearing huge platinum blond wigs teased sky high, tight dresses or vintage jumpsuits with giant bras we found in the garbage that we stuffed with hollowed-out Nerf footballs as our stage boobs! We were a sight to behold! Crooner Eddie Fisher, the New York Dolls' Johnny Thunders, comedian Judy Tenuta, and Billy Idol's guitarist Steve Stevens were just a few of the luminaries who'd drop in to do a guest appearance with us. Fred was a highly skilled promoter and schmoozer who could get anyone and everyone to do his bidding. He'd always manage to pepper the audience with celebs like Sydney 'Mayflower Madam' Biddle Barrows and Tiny Tim, Matt and Kevin Dillon, and columnists and photographers like Michael Musto and Patrick McMullan. He even somehow got Joey Ramone to go bowling with us.

"Driving home with Rocco from a gig one New Year's Eve in a huge snowstorm in our old car affectionately known as 'The Shitmobile'—because it was always

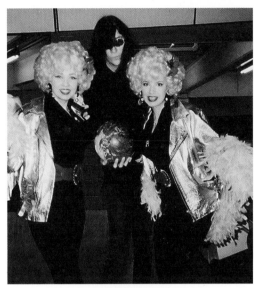

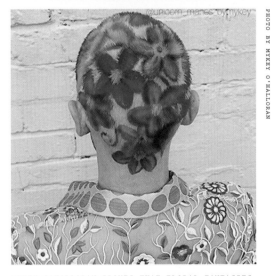

MYKEY O'HALLORAN PROVES THAT FLORAL FANTASIES AREN'T LIMITED TO LONG HAIR, USING FUCHSIA SHOCK, HOT HOT PINK, PSYCHEDELIC SUNSET, VOODOO BLUE, ATOMIC TURQUOISE, SIREN'S SONG, DEEP PURPLE DREAM, ULTRA VIOLET, MYSTIC HEATHER, ENCHANTED FOREST, GREEN ENVY, ELECTRIC LIZARD, AND ELECTRIC BANANA TO CREATE THIS GARDEN OF FLOWERS.

breaking down and looked like shit—we were pulled over by the police. Our car was missing two side windows plus the entire rear window, and snow was pouring in as the plastic bags we had taped in the windows flapped in the breeze. The heating system was broken, and somehow the air-conditioning was stuck on high and couldn't be turned off. It was so cold we could see our breath. Snowflakes danced around the beat-up interior as we drove. The cop thought we were completely nuts! He said, 'Don't you know your car is missing most of its windows?!' We were laughing so hysterically that we could hardly speak but managed to ask him politely if this was really a crime. He felt so sorry for us and let us go without a ticket and we put him on our guest list for our next gig.

"The next spring we replaced the broken windows. By the time summer rolled around, the windows were stuck shut, the AC had finally broken, and the heat kicked in full blast and couldn't be turned off! We realized later that the car must have been possessed. We should have called it Christine!"

While vibrant colors were becoming more mainstream, it was a slightly depressing time for Tish and Snooky, but they had to keep on keeping on. "The second basement we moved into had a good vibe—it had originally been the La MaMa Theatre. At one point it was also Jimi Hendrix's crash pad, since his girlfriend had lived there. We were there for three years, from 1992 to 1995, doing mostly wholesale and a little bit of retail here and there," Snooky explains. However, the new place felt like a bit of a comedown after the success of the original store. "This was even scarier than the previous location because it had extremely rickety metal steps and was really 'basement-y.' From the outside, it must have looked like

we were really out of luck at that point. But we actually weren't, because we were building a really strong wholesale business during this time."

Manic Panic had been distributing hair color that was produced in Europe. The manufacturer had guaranteed that Manic Panic would be the only company they would supply in the United States and Canada. "We were young, naive, and way too trusting. They thought we were stupid, referring to us condescendingly as 'the girls,'" says Tish. "The manufacturer was three months behind in shipping to us. All we did all day was answer the phone, apologize, and get yelled at because we had no product to ship." They soon discovered that the company was selling directly to some of their very own customers behind their backs.

Snooky adds, "Our mother was dying of cancer at the same time. It was the most miserable period of our lives."

"One day while we were in the hospital visiting our sick mother," Tish continues, "one of our employees took a small wholesale order. The next day he proudly told me that some joker paid full price and overnight shipping for our twenty best-selling colors!" The sisters soon learned that the new "customer" was a direct competitor looking to break into the vibrant hair color market. "I was like, 'What?! You just signed our death sentence!' So that guy had our twenty best colors handpicked for him!"

Sure enough, the next week at a trade show the competitor was taking orders on Manic Panic's most popular colors with his own tacky label stuck on top. He even pulled Manic Panic customers into his booth and tried to sell them what he called "Manic Color." The sisters were furious! But it got worse.

"Then this guy had the nerve to call us up and ask if we wanted to distribute *his* Manic Color!" says Tish.

ALWAYS BE A FIRST-RATE VERSION OF YOURSELF, INSTEAD OF A SECOND-RATE VERSION OF SOMEBODY ELSE.

—JUDY GARLAND

"I remember yelling, 'You CANNOT use our name! WE ARE Manic Panic. You can't call your brand Manic Color.' He replied arrogantly, 'I can call it Manic Color. I can call it Panic Color—I can call it whatever I want. I've done my homework.' I screamed, 'You'll have to talk to our lawyer about that then!' and hung up." Manic Panic's lawyer asked him to change the name. "He changed it to something totally lame," says Tish, a name "a tacky, middle-aged businessman would think was 'cool.'" And lo and behold, with his new brand, he tried to target Manic Panic's customers.

The challenges kept coming. Around the same time, Manic Panic approached a cosmetic manufacturer in Brooklyn to create an exclusive line of glitter lipsticks. "They jerked us around for a year," continues Snooky. "Right before they were finally about to deliver our goods, days before our big launch at a trade show, they said, 'Oh, we'll be seeing you at the trade show. Our good friends are exhibiting.'"

When the girls arrived at the show, it was clear why they had been kept waiting a year. Right down the aisle from Manic Panic's humble little booth loomed the Goliath booth owned by the manufacturer's "friends." They found that the company was launching what were supposed to be Manic Panic's exclusive glitter lipsticks in cheap packaging at a fraction of the price with their "friend's" company, which had a reach much larger than theirs!

"We didn't have enough business experience to even think to get an exclusive contract or anything like that—we were just so gullible," says Snooky. "But we just kept going and going like Energizer bunnies. We've always figured our way out of whatever is thrown at us. There's always going to be someone trying to screw you, but there's always a new route you can take."

Out of this frustration, the girls finally said enough was enough with importing and took matters into their own hands. Tish explains, "We tracked down the inventor of vibrant hair dyes to help us develop a line of cruelty-free, vegan hair color to our specifications, made in the USA. That was our salvation." They moved into a huge loft in Tribeca, on White Street, right down the block from their old haunt the Mudd Club, where they hung out regularly in the '80s, performing, producing theme parties, and creating art installations.

"We felt right at home in that hood," Snooky says. When they moved into White Street, Manic Panic was able to really boom because they finally had enough space to buy in bigger, bulk quantities—four thousand square feet in comparison to their two-hundred-square-foot basement. "I remember thinking, 'Oh my God, this place is so big! How are we ever going to use up all of this space?' But we filled it up right away. White Street was basically our office, showroom, and warehouse—friends and longtime customers of Manic Panic would come by to say hi or place an order."

WE [NEW YORK CITY] ARE THE AMERICAN CRADLE OF PUNK ROCK, HOME TO A VERY COLORFUL CAST OF CHARACTERS, AND A PLACE WHERE LIFE IS SOMETIMES MANIC-PANICKED. THEREFORE, IT'S NO SURPRISE THAT OUR RESIDENTS HAVE BECOME SO FOND OF YOUR HAIR DYE, CLOTHING, AND COSMETICS.

—MICHAEL BLOOMBERG,
former mayor of NYC on the
occasion of Manic Panic's
30th anniversary

With their cosmetic and hair dye shades, produced by a newer, and more reliable, manufacturing company, Manic Panic was an unstoppable, colorful force in a rather lackluster beauty industry. Tish fondly reflects, "We got our first big delivery right when we moved—huge pallet loads full of Manic Panic domestically made hair dye! We couldn't believe it."

It was an amazing feeling after many years of being at the mercy of an unreliable supplier. At that point, Tish and Snooky knew what they wanted to create and what needed to be improved. More importantly, because of the time spent managing customer service firsthand, they knew exactly what their customers wanted.

"We worked so hard with various chemists to improve longevity in color," says Tish. "Based on customer feedback, we just kept refining the formula throughout the years to perfect it as much as we could. We're still improving to this day, keeping ahead by evolving as soon as there are new technological advances. An excellent example is Manic Panic Pro, which uses new technology and innovation to allow professional colorists to incorporate techniques that were previously too difficult and time consuming."

Manic Panic began locally manufacturing their top twelve colors, which includes shades still produced, such as Vampire Red, Shocking Blue, Green Envy, Ultra Violet, Hot Hot Pink, Infra Red, and Sunshine. The first beauty company to give all of its colors unusual names, Manic Panic quickly started adding more and more new shades.

"Whenever someone famous, in a band or otherwise, dyed their hair a certain color—like when Kurt Cobain dyed his hair with Hot Hot Pink, or when Cyndi Lauper dyed hers yellow using a mix of Sunshine and Electric Banana, or when Flea from Red Hot Chili Peppers did his in Atomic Turquoise—sales would spike," Tish says. "We'd have to start producing extra stock

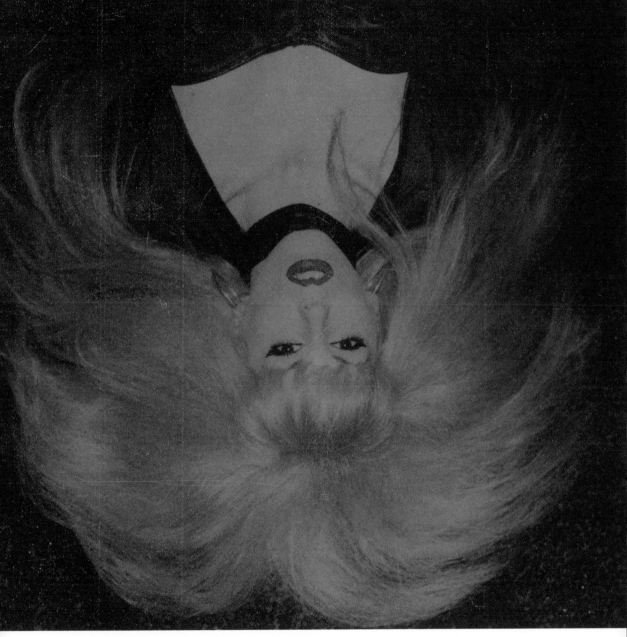

MANIC PANIC DYEHARD GYDA GASH IN THE EARLY '90S.
PHOTO BY LEONARD DRINDELL

of a certain color because the trend would
take off like a bat outta hell."

As Manic Panic provided a brand-new
generation with its hair color, business
continued to grow during the '90s. With new
trends, bands, and hairstyles emerging,
Tish and Snooky were ready to dive headfirst
into the next millennium of beauty.

PRETTY
IN **PINK,**
ISN'T
SHE

COLOR GUIDE

(OR HE)
(OR THEY)?

MANIC PANIC CLASSIC HIGH VOLTAGE, AMPLIFIED, AND PROFESSIONAL COLORS

CLEO ROSE *(NAMED AFTER OUR DEAR FRIEND AND MENTOR)*	COTTON CANDY PINK	FUCHSIA SHOCK	HOT HOT PINK	PRETTY FLAMINGO	PUSSYCAT PINK

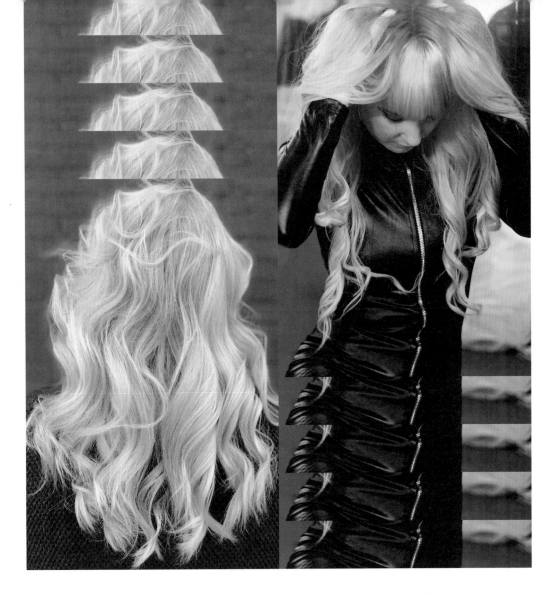

TWO VERY DIFFERENT LOOKS
CAN BE ATTAINED BY HAVING
DIFFERENT BASE COLORS.
ON THE LEFT, CORINNE PELTIER
USED MANIC PANIC SILVER
STILETTO TO PLATINUM-IZE
OUR CREAMTONE FLEURS DU MAL.
ON THE RIGHT, MANIC PANIC
PRO IS USED TO BLEND THE
COLORS TOGETHER TO CREATE A
BRIGHT AND DYNAMIC LOOK.

PHOTO (LEFT) BY CORINNE PELTIER;
PHOTO (RIGHT) BY ALESSANDRO BIANCHERI

As seen on everyone from Kurt Cobain to Kate Moss, pink hair was a huge color trend in the 1990s, and it's no surprise why: Pink is one of those shades that looks good on everyone, no matter gender, skin tone, or hair texture. Like yellow, it's an easy color to transition to if you're starting from blond, especially if you're trying to remedy a brassy blond job. Here, we chat with UK-based hair colorist Steven Austin on how to rock a pink look.

"Pink hair is so eye-catching, and I think it's so punk due to its juxtaposition, since pink is generally considered 'girly' and soft. To have pink hair and yet not be anything that's generally associated with the color is what makes it so punk!

In 1978...I was fourteen?...I purchased Hot Pink Hair Dye from my friends Tish and Snooky at Manic Panic NYC (so I've known them for forty years!). I bleached my hair white, dyed it Hot Pink, maybe it was Shocking Pink (not exactly sure of the title), went to school (seventh or eighth grade)...and was immediately ejected into detention and quickly kicked out of school. I believe I was the first one to ever go to school with Manic Panic hair color.... I was treated like Frankenstein's monster. (Funny, though, now it's NOT looked at twice and has become the norm! FINALLY!!!!!) Next, the principal made me promise NOT to come to graduation with pink hair (my hair was blond at the time). Ready for more Manic Panic, I promised...and went to eighth-grade graduation with pink hair, a pink suit, and New Rock shoes on!!! They refused to give me my diploma, so I sat on the stage and proceeded to give the principal the finger. It was the first of many riots I would incite in my future music career!! Hahahahaha!! Google it!

"PUNKED PINK PUPIL PROVOKES PRINCIPAL."

STYLIST STEVEN
AUSTIN CREATED
THIS MAGNIFICENT
HOT PINK MANE
USING TWO OF OUR
PROFESSIONAL
COLORS, DIVINE WINE
AND PUSSYCAT PINK.

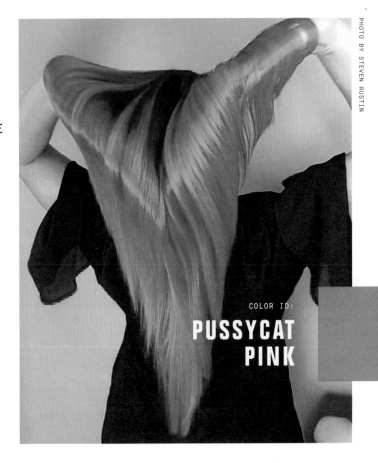

COLOR ID:

PUSSYCAT
PINK

"For those new to vivid colors such as pink, my immediate advice is: Go for it! It can literally be life changing. My clients tell me all the time when they make the switch to a new color like pink, they feel like themselves again. People come up and talk to them more, they make new friends, their confidence grows—it's the best. Naturally there will be people out there who don't like your hair color, but the best advice I can give is to flip that new hair, stare them down, and walk on with confidence. Remember, their hair color can be found in dirt—yours can be seen in rainbows!

"The key to beginning to go to pink is to prelighten hair to a nice, light blond first, while determining what shade of pink you'd want to achieve. For pinks, I rarely use just one color. I personally love using Fuchsia Shock as a root shadow, then applying Hot Hot Pink or Cleo Rose on the mid lengths, and then Cotton Candy Pink on the ends. Skin tone and face shape doesn't really come into play with vivid colors like pink; I think it's all about attitude! I'd recommend leaving the pink hair dye on for about as long as it takes to watch a rerun of *RuPaul's Drag Race*—so about forty-five minutes.

"After, you'll want to rinse the hair in cool water, and then one final cold rinse. I prefer cold rinses when working with hair colors such as pink because they prevent any color leaking and really preserve the color's longevity. Afterward, dry your hair and then hopefully squeal with delight and take a million selfies to show it off!"

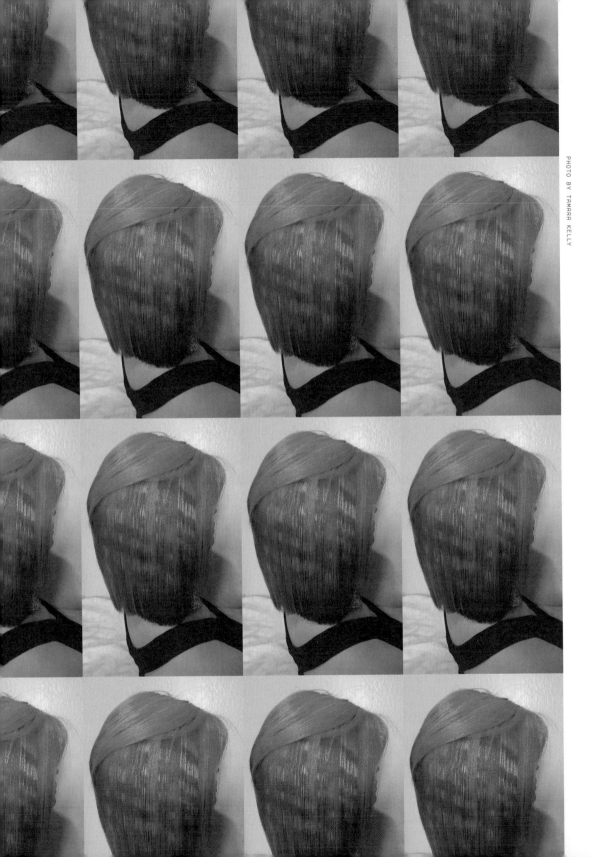

TAMARA KELLY MADE
OUR HOT HOT PINK
HIGH VOLTAGE
CLASSIC CREAM POP
EVEN MORE WITH
UNDER LAYERS OF
ULTRA VIOLET.

COLOR ID:
PUSSYCAT
PINK

COLOR ID:
ULTRA VIOLET

I PUT MANIC PANIC IN MY HAIR TO MAKE THE TIPS PINK. THAT WAS A BIG HIT IN MY FAMILY. MAMA WAS REALLY COOL BECAUSE OF THAT.

—HEIDI KLUM

IT'S A **BLUE,** BLUE SUMMER

COLOR GUIDE

MANIC PANIC CLASSIC HIGH VOLTAGE, AMPLIFIED, AND PROFESSIONAL COLORS

AFTER MIDNIGHT	ATOMIC TURQUOISE	BAD BOY BLUE	BLUE MOON	BLUE BAYOU	CELESTINE BLUE
BLUE STEEL	MERMAID	ROCKABILLY BLUE	SHOCKING BLUE	VOODOO BLUE	BLUE VELVET

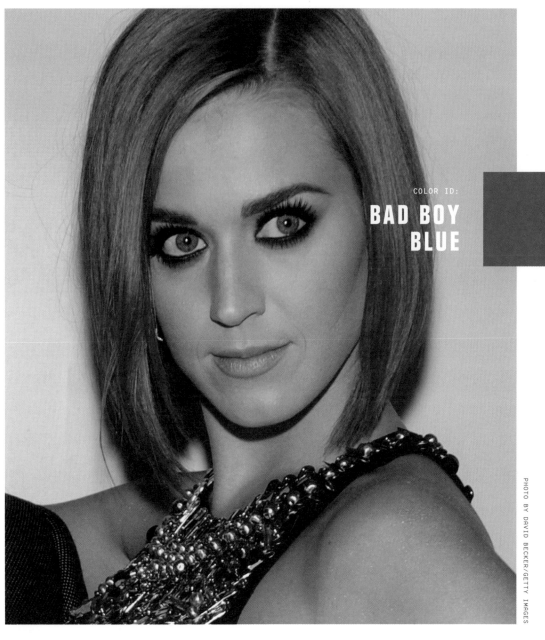

PHOTO BY DAVID BECKER/GETTY IMAGES

Gwen Stefani of No Doubt rocked blue locks on the red carpet of the MTV VMAs in 1998 while sporting a matching fuzzy blue rhinestone-encrusted bra top, making blue one of the iconic colors of the '90s. "Our friend Kelly, who was a roadie and guitar tech, would keep No Doubt living in color with a constant supply of Manic Panic for the whole band," Tish recalls.

CHECK OUT KATY PERRY SPORTING OUR BAD BOY BLUE CLASSIC CREAM AT THE OPENING OF 1 OAK IN LAS VEGAS.

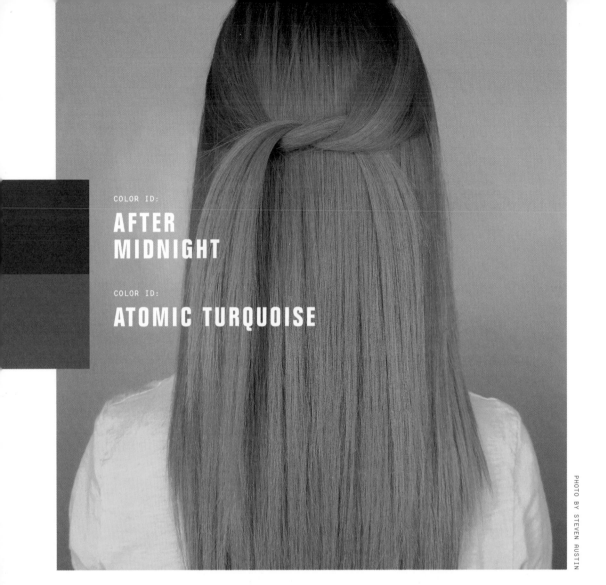

COLOR ID:

AFTER MIDNIGHT

COLOR ID:

ATOMIC TURQUOISE

Blue hair was also spotted on the heads of Billie Joe Armstrong of Green Day as well as designer Todd Oldham during the '90s.

We spoke with hair colorist Mykey O'Halloran on the beauty of blue hair and its moment in the '90s.

"I love bringing color into people's worlds, as well as the freedom of expression, empowerment, and confidence for everyone—that's what Manic Panic colors give to people. I had a client recently that had always wanted blue hair; she was a natural brunette with beautiful olive skin. Depending on what hair color you're starting out with, everyone will have a different hair history to begin with. For some, the hair may require two bleaches in one sitting to get it light enough to even apply a blue hue—for others, if they already have a prelightened or natural blond, then half of the work is already done.

STYLIST STEVEN AUSTIN CREATED THESE TURQUOISE TRESSES USING AFTER MIDNIGHT, VOODOO FOREST, RAVEN, ATOMIC TURQUOISE, AND SERPENTINE GREEN.

WELL, LET ME TELL YOU, I HAVE EXPERIENCE WITH MANIC PANIC. I HAD JUST DONE MY LAST TOUR—AND THIS WAS PRE–KATY PERRY—BUT I HAD THAT BLUE HAIR THAT'S IN THE MOVIE (*KELLY & CAL*). IT WAS THIS AMAZING AQUA COLOR. IT'S THE COLOR OF THE COSMIC SEA IN *THE LITTLE MERMAID*. THEY NEED TO MAKE A COLOR CALLED COSMIC SEA.

—JULIETTE LEWIS

PHOTO BY MYKEY O'HALLORAN

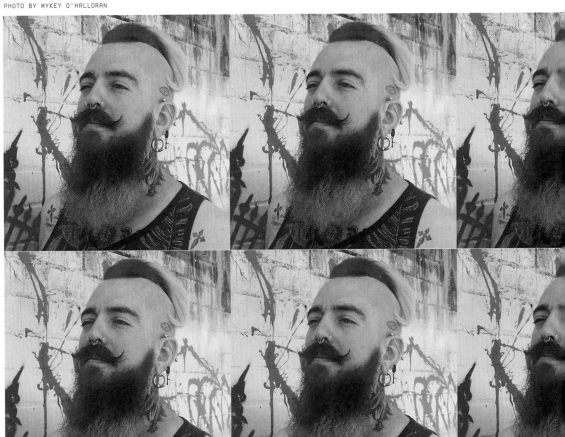

MANIC PANIC BRAND AMBASSADOR MYKEY O'HALLORAN CREATED THIS MERMAN MELT USING ELECTRIC BANANA, VOODOO BLUE, AND CELESTINE BLUE.

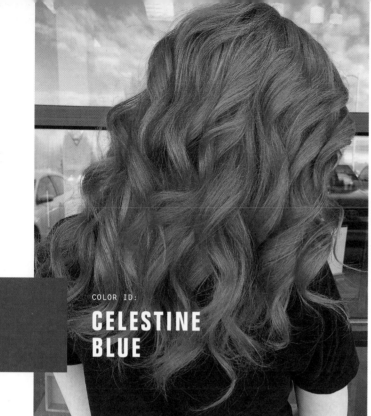

COLOR ID:

CELESTINE BLUE

BRAND AMBASSADOR ANGELA BECKER USED CELESTINE BLUE AND VELVET VIOLET TO CREATE THIS BEAUTIFUL BLUE-VIOLET-HUED HAIR STYLE.

"Personally, I love using Manic Panic's Celestine Blue and Blue Velvet; both are from their Professional Gel Semi-Permanent Hair Color line—they give the best coverage I have ever seen from a blue dye. I use both of them quite frequently because they're also super long-lasting. Since they're both deeper shades of blue, I like to use them both at the roots and then melt them into variations of Voodoo Blue on the ends, which is a more turquoise shade of blue. I also suggest Blue Moon, After Midnight, Shocking Blue, and Rockabilly Blue—those are my favorite royal blue shades in the classic line. These shades are also great on coverage because they're so highly pigmented, so make sure you wear gloves if you're using them at home!

"After prelightening the base canvas to blond, I like to apply the Manic Panic dyes on damp hair, since it helps with color blending. If the hair is extremely damaged, then I'll do some kind of hair treatment to help restore and repair hair after lifting it with bleach so it stays in the healthiest condition. I never pick a specific color based on a client's skin tone—I would give anyone any color that they asked for. I don't really believe in warm or cool colors based on skin tone. More so, I think about brightness and intensity, and what level the color sits on. For example, with my brunette client going full-on blue after a double bleach process, choosing a combo like Celestine Blue and Blue Velvet adds depth to the color. My client will feel like they have a deep shade at the roots, which will surprisingly feel more natural to them because it isn't a fluorescent or lighter shade of blue at the roots.

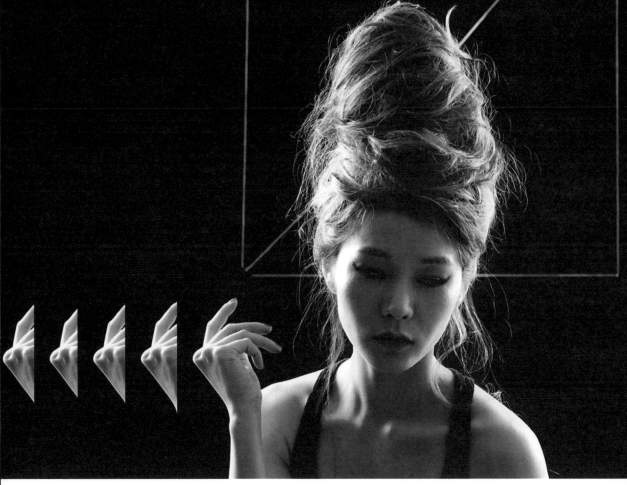

STYLIST MAISAWA
MASAMITSU CREATED
AN ARCHITECTURAL
BEEHIVE USING A
MEDLEY OF MANIC
PANIC BLUES.

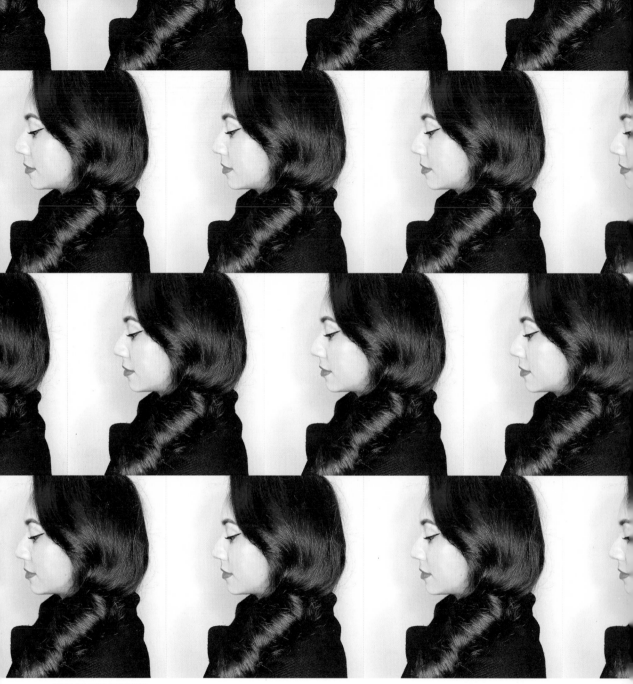

STYLIST DOUG
MACINTOSH CREATED
THESE COBALT CURLS
USING BALAYAGE
WITH CELESTINE
BLUE OVER IT.

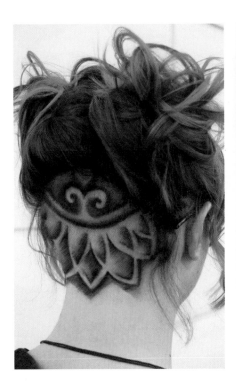

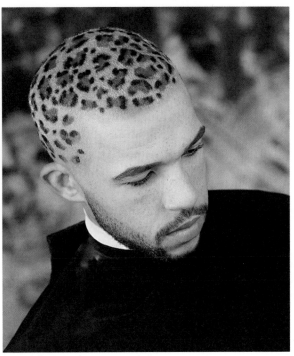

"I recommend leaving the Manic Panic color on for about twenty to thirty minutes to process, and then rinsing out with cool water. I also always recommend that my clients wash their hair with cool water at home to help keep the Manic Panic dyes in to ensure longevity, since their classic range is designed to last up to eight weeks, while their professional line can last up to forty washes. The last step would be to blow-dry hair, starting in the front so you can see what your new hair color looks like, since wet hair and dry hair look completely different when it's a new color!

"When I think of blue-hair icons in the 1990s, I think of Gwen Stefani, which at the time was such a statement when she did it and such an iconic signature color for her in her career—not everyone was taking hair-color risks like that back then. I also think of Marge Simpson and Milhouse Van Houten, both characters in *The Simpsons*, around this same time—both female and male characters wearing the same shade of blue, which no other character had, was always pretty cool to me. I once dyed a client's hair with Bad Boy Blue and he told me he got called a Smurf on the street after I did his hair. He politely made a correction back to advise the insulter that Smurfs have white hats, and their skin is what's blue—which is a great response!"

ABOVE LEFT

CHECK OUT THIS INTRICATE UNDERCUT BY ANGELA SKULLPTURES USING ENCHANTED FOREST AND ELECTRIC LIZARD.

PHOTO BY ANGELA SKULLPTURES

ABOVE RIGHT

STYLIST SHAROON TYLER CREATED THIS BEAUTIFUL BLUE LEOPARD PRINT USING RAVEN AND PASTEL-IZED BAD BOY BLUE.

PHOTO BY SHAROON TYLER

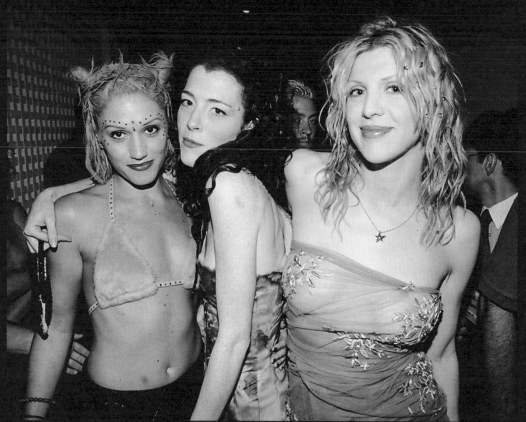

PHOTO BY JEFF KRAVITZ/GETTY IMAGES

"Being in a band, you can wear whatever you want—
it's like an excuse for

HALLOWEEN EVERY DAY."

—GWEN STEFANI

HOW TO AVOID A MESS

Dyeing your hair at home can often be messy, but the following tips should help:

- WEAR OLD CLOTHES, OR USE TISH'S TIP OF MAKING A GARBAGE BAG INTO A DRESS, AND USE OLD TOWELS YOU DON'T MIND STAINING.

- PLACE PETROLEUM JELLY AROUND YOUR HAIRLINE, EARS, AND NECK TO PROTECT YOUR SKIN FROM BEING STAINED. BE CAREFUL NOT TO GET ANY OF THE PETROLEUM JELLY ON YOUR HAIR, AS THE DYE WILL NOT PENETRATE IF IT DOES.

- PROTECT THE FLOOR AND ANY WORK SURFACES WITH NEWSPAPERS, TRASH BAGS, OR OLD TOWELS YOU DON'T MIND STAINING. FYI: MANIC PANIC MAKES BLACK TOWELS SPECIFICALLY FOR THIS PURPOSE.

- ALWAYS WEAR PLASTIC GLOVES, EVEN WHEN WORKING WITH LIGHTER DYES, TO AVOID COLORING YOUR HANDS.

- USE MANIC PANIC DYE AWAY WIPES TO REMOVE ANY DYE STAINS THAT MAY OCCUR ON SKIN.

- RINSE HAIR IN A STAINLESS-STEEL SINK IF POSSIBLE, AS SOME COLORS MAY TEMPORARILY STAIN LIGHT SINKS OR BATHTUBS.

- IF YOU DO GET THE HAIR COLOR ON YOUR SINK OR OTHER SURFACES, SPRAY BLEACH WORKS GREAT FOR REMOVAL!

"Our friend/bass player Steve Mach from the '90s band Skin N' Bones always advised anyone about to color their hair to wait to get to a hotel room, or else do it at a friend's house!"

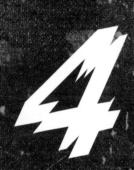

4

ENTERING THE MILLENNIUM IN STYLE:

THE RETURN OF PUNK ROCK GIRLS

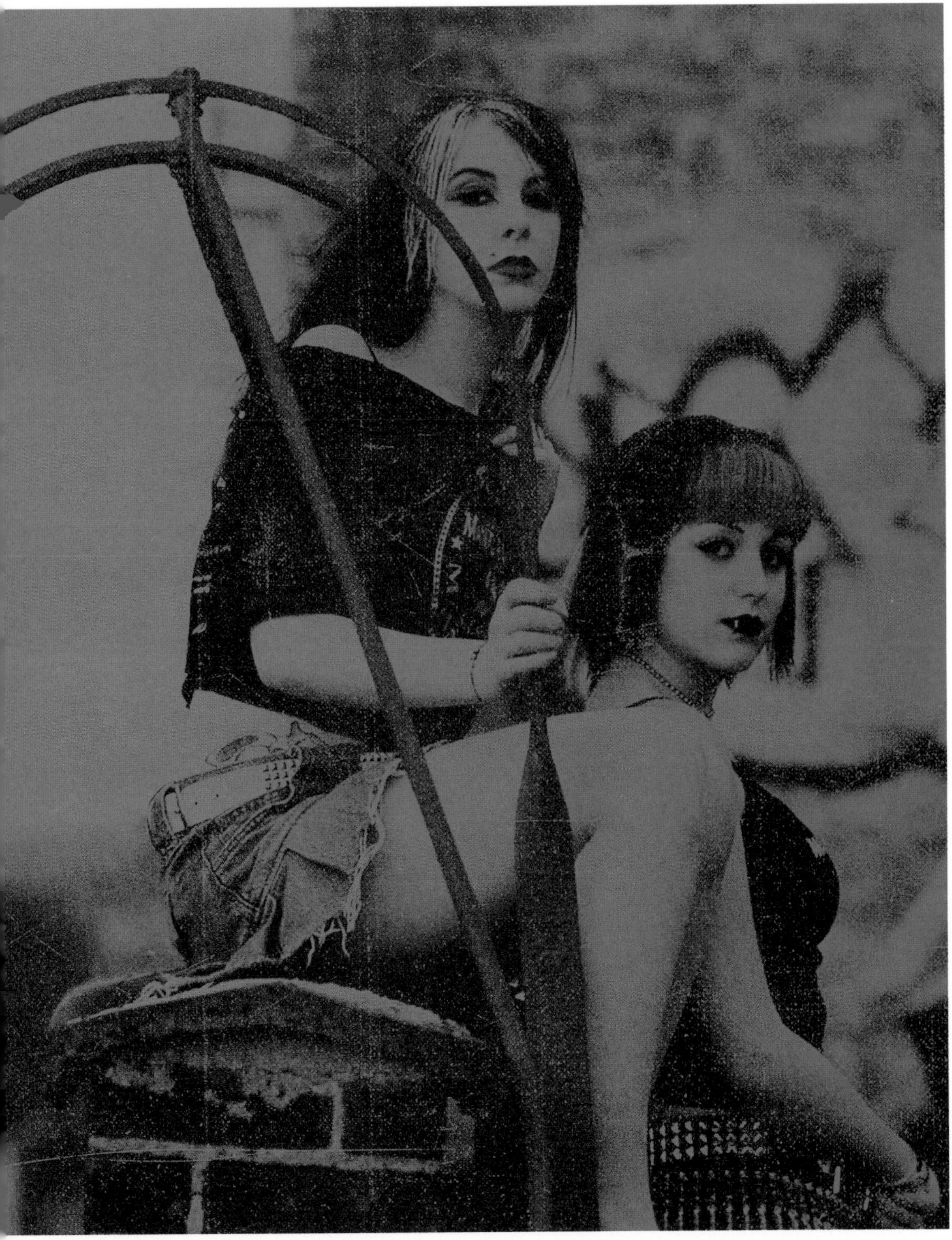

MILLENNIUM GIRLS ON THE ROOF OF MANIC PANIC HEADQUARTERS

PHOTO BY PETER PERENYI

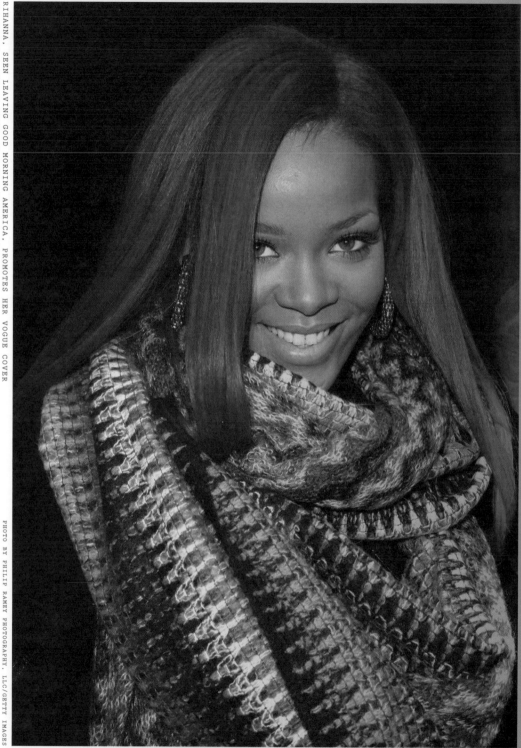

RIHANNA, SEEN LEAVING GOOD MORNING AMERICA, PROMOTES HER VOGUE COVER FEATURING A SECRET BLEND OF MANIC PANIC CLASSIC COLORS.

PHOTO BY PHILIP RAMEY PHOTOGRAPHY, LLC/GETTY IMAGES

ountdown to a new millennium! Times were changing, but some things never change: Gentrification had once again reared its ugly head, making rents skyrocket, uprooting them from their White Street location.

"The neighborhood got hot and the landlord grew cold, wanting to quadruple our rent. He wanted architects, lawyers, and virtual companies to move in and for us to move out," Snooky remembers. "It was a horrible feeling because we were displaced after spending so much time and money building out the space and really making it our own."

Tish chimes in: "They didn't even want to negotiate the lease with us. We ended up moving out of Manhattan at the end of 1999."

Manic Panic rang in the new millennium at a new location in Long Island City, Queens, which was four times the size of White Street. Once again they thought, *How are we ever going to use all this space?* But once again, they did.

The sisters hit the ground running, frantically trying to keep up with the increasing demand. "We had barely enough time to set up the new space before we started shipping. We couldn't even finish unpacking! In fact, we still haven't finished unpacking, even after almost twenty years," says Tish with a laugh. "There's still a treasure trove of vintage merch from the first store on St. Marks Place sitting somewhere in the back of our warehouse. Someday we'll have the time to unearth it all. Stay tuned for our Manic Panic tag sale!"

The music trends of grunge, alternative, and riot grrrl were now being supplemented with genres of emo, pop punk, metal, and hard-core. This shift was in part thanks to the popularity of social media platforms, starting with Myspace being introduced to a younger and more tech-savvy generation.

And with this sudden, worldwide connection came the birth of the social media influencer. Internet celebrities— dubbed "scene queens"—became known for dyeing their hair in various Manic Panic colors, including Jeffree Star, Audrey Kitching, Kiki Kannibal, Raquel Reed, and Hanna Beth. Their new and unique style was obsessed over and copied. Taking direct cues from punk rockers in the '70s and mixing it with a more modern glam, they rocked black and purple hair, raccoon hair stripes, and teased-out roots.

Manic Panic sales grew with this wave, going from the sidewalk to the catwalk, adding even more products into stores such as Hot Topic and Sally Beauty.

GIRLS GOIN' GLOBAL:
AIN'T NO STOPPIN' US NOW!

"Going global meant going with our gut. One of our trusted business advisors cautioned us that expanding overseas would be a really bad move. 'Play in your own backyard!' we were told. We could've been good little girls and listened, but no freakin' way!" Tish says with a laugh.

"Ever since we were little kids, we were fascinated by other cultures and collected dolls and knick-knacks from all around the world," adds Snooky. "We were always attracted to the kids in school from other countries; we wanted to understand their customs, taste their food, and listen to their music. Our goal was to travel the world, and as adults we weren't about to let anyone get in our way."

Without any international experience or know-how, the sisters jumped in with both feet, exhibiting at trade shows in the UK, Germany, and Italy to start. As in the United States, Manic Panic was most popular with the alternative, clubby trade shows and events geared toward nightlife and extreme fashion.

"One of our favorite shows was the Night Wave trade show in Italy, which started in the late afternoon and went until ten or eleven at night," says Tish. "Then everyone went to dinner and then out to the clubs until dawn, many sleeping on the beach. They'd come back the next afternoon and do it all over again."

They had a totally different experience at CosmoProf in Italy, where most of the attendees and exhibitors, not to mention show management, didn't know what to make of them or their products. "They looked at us as if we were from Mars," Snooky says, laughing. Their booth décor one year nearly got them banned from the show. "Black lace and velvet were draped throughout and we were dressed in our usual Gothy-glam drag topped with rainbow-colored hair. Our booth was the scandal of the show! We were told that it looked like a bordello and that unless we toned it down, we'd never be allowed back. We grudgingly complied the next year, only to find that half the booths at the show looked like ours did the year before!"

Defying conventional advice and stepping out of their comfort zone gave Manic Panic early entry into the global market. "It was always our dream that Manic Panic products would be available everywhere on the planet and beyond. That dream is coming true. Forty countries and counting! We hope to become the first alternative hair color on Mars."

OPPOSITE
FRENCH STYLISTS DEBORAH DARDI
AND OLIVIA IANNARELLI
CREATED THESE DUELING BOBS
FOR A FASHION SHOOT BY
ALESSANDRO BIANCHERI.

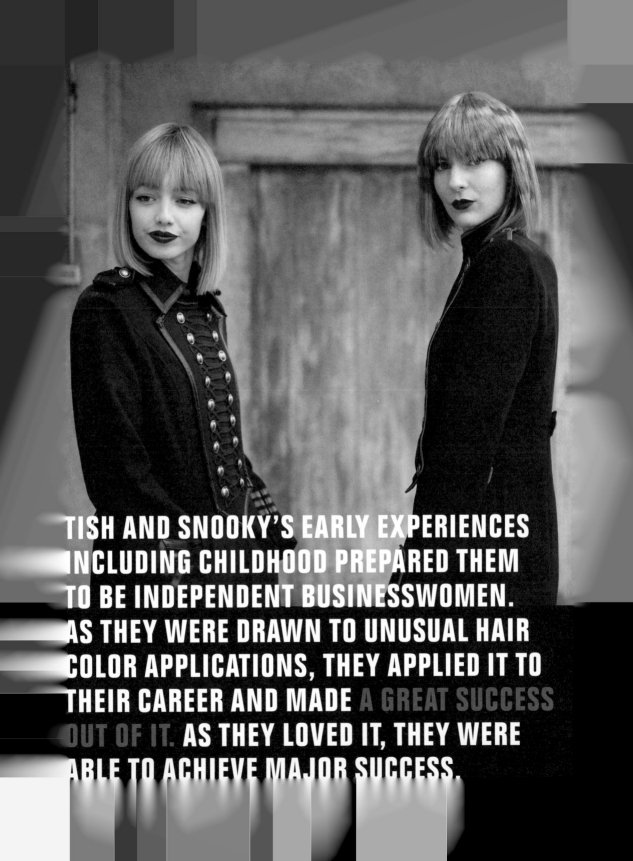

TISH AND SNOOKY'S EARLY EXPERIENCES INCLUDING CHILDHOOD PREPARED THEM TO BE INDEPENDENT BUSINESSWOMEN. AS THEY WERE DRAWN TO UNUSUAL HAIR COLOR APPLICATIONS, THEY APPLIED IT TO THEIR CAREER AND MADE A GREAT SUCCESS OUT OF IT. AS THEY LOVED IT, THEY WERE ABLE TO ACHIEVE MAJOR SUCCESS.

Tish and Snooky continued developing new products. "When we first moved to Long Island City, we launched our own line of colorizing shampoos, which deposited color while cleaning hair," says Tish. "It was formulated to be very low sudsing, because bubbles can remove color from hair. People didn't understand the low suds because they were used to bubbles. They thought that if it didn't bubble, it didn't clean. It freaked people out—it worked great but was twenty years before its time."

After visiting their friend and lawyer Alan Harris in Venice Beach, the girls were inspired to take another leap of faith, this time across the country in California. "We opened up our Venice Beach store around 2006," says Snooky, "in an area that reminded us of a beach version of St. Marks Place before it got all commercialized—it had this really amazing cutting-edge, punk, hippie vibe about it, with a touch of danger once the sun went down."

After years in wholesale, the sisters really wanted to dive back into retail and get back in touch with their customers. Opening a store in New York was out of the question because real estate was so expensive. "I remember calling around to get prices. They would quote me the monthly rent, which I thought was the yearly rent. Even for yearly, I thought that was expensive!" Snooky laughs. "It was impossible in New York, but Venice Beach was possible, so we did that for a while." They found a space that was once a cabana in Charlie Chaplin's beach house, which felt right.

The store's clientele grew and included actors such as Kirsten Dunst and Forest Whitaker, Lady Gaga's hair stylist, and many more celebrities. They also opened a salon in the same courtyard upstairs, which had breathtaking views of the ocean.

With all its appeal, the Venice Beach storefront was somewhat hard for customers to find and it was seasonal, so they moved to Melrose Avenue, and history repeated itself. They pioneered a down-and-out neighborhood, and five years later, the landlord refused to renew their lease.

"Unfortunately, the rise of corporate chains has forced out independent brick-and-mortar boutiques. We continue to do an amazing amount of business on the West Coast. While we loved meeting our customers face-to-face, now we meet them in cyberspace thanks to social media's meteoric rise," says Tish.

VENICE BEACH AND MELROSE DYEHARDS

Alexis Arquette (actress and activist)

Alice Cooper (singer)

Ana Gasteyer (comedian)

Carmen Electra (actress)

Cindy Dunaway (costume designer)

Daniel Ash (musician)

Dennis Dunaway (musician)

Forest Whitaker (actor) and his daughter

Groovie Mann (musician)

Kirsten Dunst (actress)

Lars Ulrich (musician)

Patricia Arquette (actress)

Sune Rose Wagner (singer)

Tallulah Willis (actress)

Texas Terri (singer)

Yelawolf (singer)

COLORING DREADLOCKS

Colorist Nico Norris enjoyed playing with different looks for her dreadlocks: "When I cut my dreads off, I cut one in half. There were rings of different colors inside, because when you're applying color, it mainly stays on the outer layer. I personally never saturated that intensely because it takes so much time to rinse dreads." A few words of advice:

- Don't bleach your dreads too often if you plan on growing them out. They seem strong but can't take multiple bleach sessions.

- After bleaching your dreads, make sure to lather the shampoo extremely well. Rinsing is even more important, to get ALL that bleach out. Having dreads is like having sponges for hair, so you have to just keep wringing them out and rinsing until there's no more color or soap.

STYLIST MAISAWA MASAMITSU CREATED THESE TECHNICOLOR DREADLOCKS USING GREEN ENVY, PILLAR-BOX RED, AND OUR FLASH LIGHTNING BLEACH KITS.

PHOTO BY MAISAWA MASAMITSU

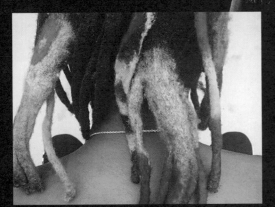

STYLIST PALMA WRIGHT CREATED THIS RAINBOW DREADLOCK LOOK USING A RAINBOW OF MANIC PANIC CLASSIC HIGH VOLTAGE HAIR COLORS.

PHOTO BY PALMA WRIGHT

BACK IN
BLACK

COLOR GUIDE

MANIC PANIC CLASSIC HIGH VOLTAGE, AMPLIFIED, AND PROFESSIONAL COLORS

| ALIEN GREY | RAVEN | BLUE STEEL | SILVER STILETTO | SMOKESCREEN | AMETHYST ASHES |

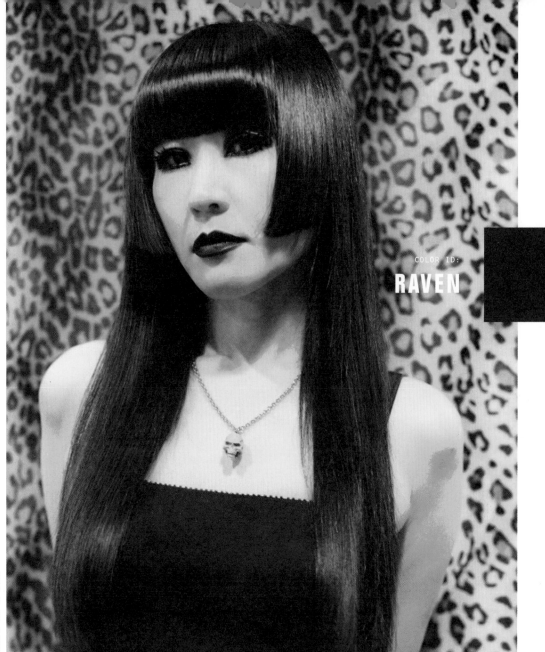

COLOR ID:
RAVEN

Black may be the most New York color of all time, perfect for the 2000 generation of emo, Goth, and hard-core kids alike. Feeling angsty? Black is the perfect color to express it. Everyone from Gerard Way, Kelly Osbourne, and Avril Lavigne were rocking onyx hues on their tresses—and even the most unexpected, anti-punk celebs like Christina Aguilera and Nicole Richie were spotted with black stripes at the ends of their hair.

MANIC PANIC
STYLIST AYUMI
MITSUISHI IN HER
TRADEMARK RAVEN
CLASSIC CREAM.

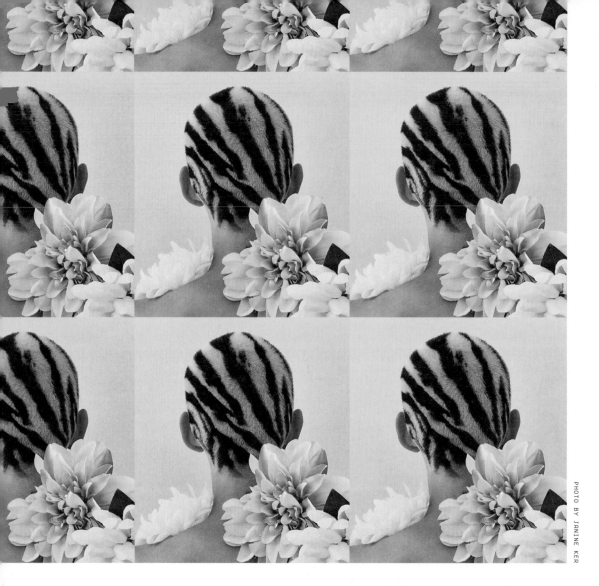

PHOTO BY JANINE KER

STYLIST JANINE
KER CREATED THIS
AMAZING ZEBRA-
PRINT HAIR STYLE,
USING RAVEN
CLASSIC CREAM
AND VIRGIN SNOW
TONER.

Colorist Ayumi Mitsuishi has always been a fan of Manic Panic Raven, saying, "My image is very heavy metal/punk, and it helps keep my look very sexy and cool. Growing up in Japan, everyone has black hair, but it isn't as deep as Manic Panic Raven. Naturally Japanese hair can be black but with a brown/orange undertone. When I use Raven, it makes it more mysterious and gives me a deep, dark color."

Ayumi also uses Raven to create a leopard print on hair, offering this advice: "Dry the hair completely after prelightening, which will make the hair easier to paint. Use a makeup brush to paint more detailed spots. My favorite is an eye shadow brush, which is small enough and the soft bristles allow me to paint smoothly. It is important to leave the Raven on the hair until color is completely dry. If the color is dry, it will not bleed when rinsed out."

"*Rocky Horror Picture Show* is still, to this day, one of my favorite movies of all time," Kelly Osbourne told *HotSpots!* magazine. "I loved the makeup. If you look really closely at the 'Time Warp,' you'll see

WHERE I GET ALL MY HAIR COLORS FROM."

PURPLE

HAZE, ALL IN MY HAIR

COLOR GUIDE

MANIC PANIC CLASSIC HIGH VOLTAGE, AMPLIFIED, AND PROFESSIONAL COLORS

AMETHYST ASHES	DEEP PURPLE DREAM	ELECTRIC AMETHYST	LIE LOCKS	VELVET VIOLET	
MYSTIC HEATHER	PLUM PASSION	PURPLE HAZE	ULTRA VIOLET	VIOLET NIGHT	LOVE POWER PURPLE

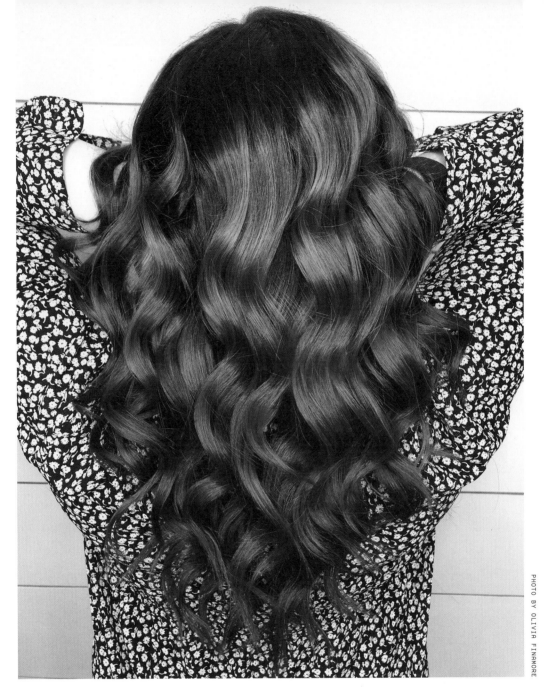

OLIVIA FINAMORE
USED EVERY
SHADE OF PURPLE
IMAGINABLE TO
CREATE THIS
AMAZING LOOK.

Purple hair dye was also extremely popular during the early 2000s, thanks to the Myspace and Hot Topic influences. One star who helped kick it off was Lil' Kim, whose purple hair matched her barely there jumpsuit at the 1999 MTV VMAs. Here, we talk with hair colorist Lucy Gonzalez, who gives us the 411 on all things purple!

WHETHER YOU WEAR YOUR HAIR CURLY OR
STRAIGHT, IT ALL LOOKS GREAT IN PURPLES.
LEFT TO RIGHT: HAIR BY STYLISTS JAVIERA
CAMACHO AND VALENTINA ARAVENA.

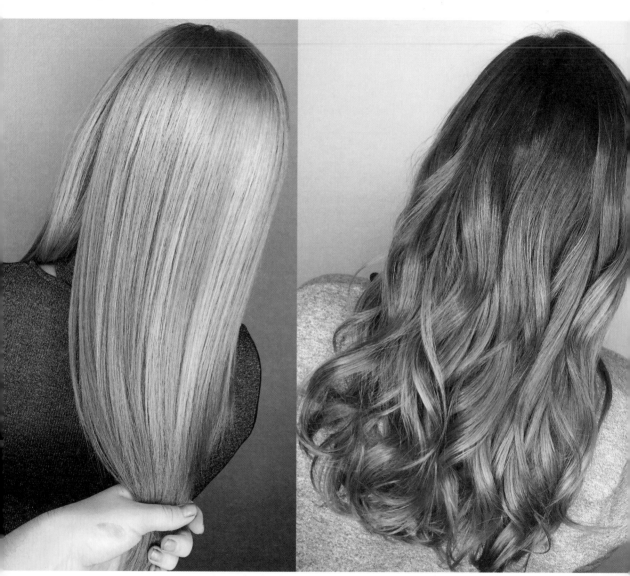

PHOTOS BY (LEFT) JAVIERA CAMACHO
AND (RIGHT) VALENTINA ARAVENA

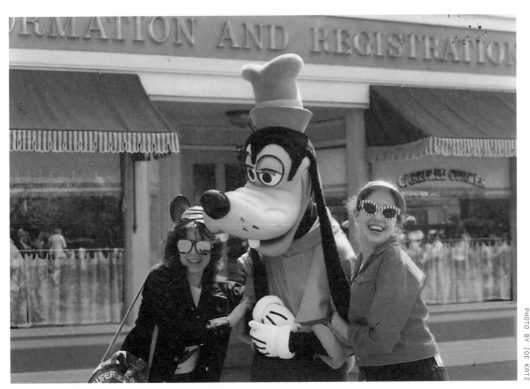

TISH AND SNOOKY AT DISNEYLAND WITH GOOFY, WHO REMARKED IN A TOTAL GOOFY VOICE, "P-URRRRPLE HAIR??!" "NO, IT'S FUCHSIA YOU IDIOT!" IT WAS RARE BACK IN THE '70s, BUT BY THE 2000s IT WAS SEEN ON LIL' KIM!

"When a client of mine wants to go a vivid color like purple, I do let them know that there will be looks. Many people may stop them on the street to ask them questions about it. When someone takes the leap to do a full color, they tell me they've never felt better—it's like a magical-mermaid-unicorn type of feeling!"

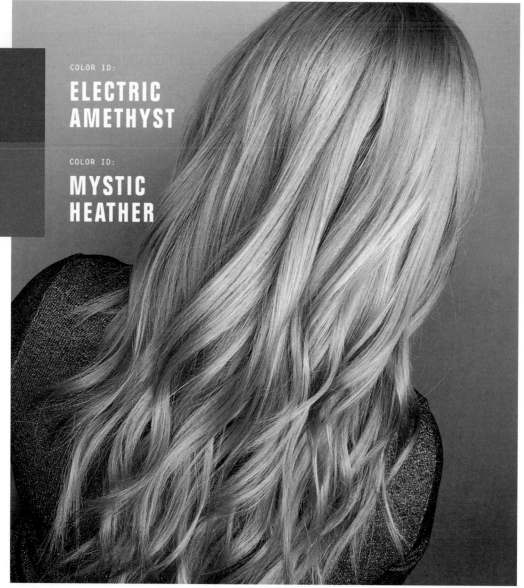

PHOTOS BY JAVIERA CAMACHO

COLOR ID:

ELECTRIC AMETHYST

COLOR ID:

MYSTIC HEATHER

STYLIST JAVIERA CAMACHO CREATED THIS BEAUTIFUL OMBRÉ OF LIGHT TO DARK PURPLE USING PASTELIZED ELECTRIC AMETHYST AND MYSTIC HEATHER.

"To properly achieve the right shade of purple, all you have to do is lift the hair to a platinum blond, which doesn't have to be perfect. You'll also want to tone the hair, or change the shade, to give it more of a cooler-purple shade or a more pastel-purple shade. Toning is ideal to get all the yellow in the lifted hair out. But if you're doing a darker purple, then leaving the bleached hair slightly yellow is totally fine!

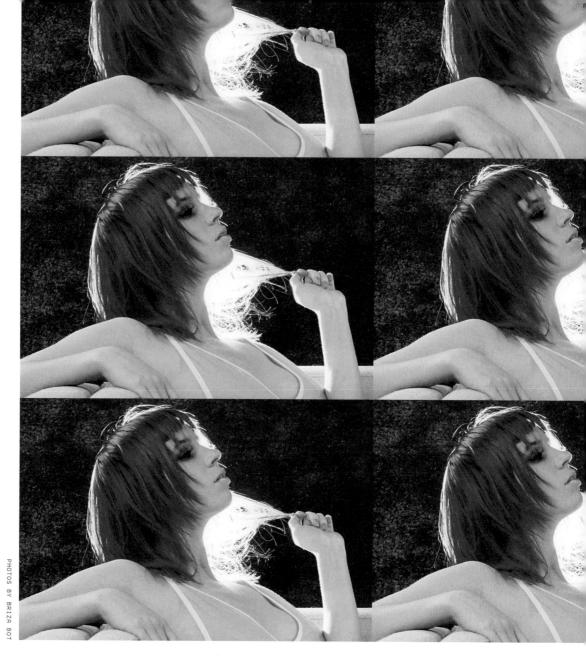

"Manic Panic has bleach kits, so if you want to do this at home, you can use their 30 or 40 volume kit. But depending on the shade of purple you're going for, you need to watch how light your ends are turning. Never, ever bleach on clean hair—it's preferable to bleach dirty hair so that the oils on the scalp can protect the head from any scalp damage.

THIS MODEL LOOKS STUNNING IN THIS PURPLE HAZE AND LIE LOCKS BLEND.

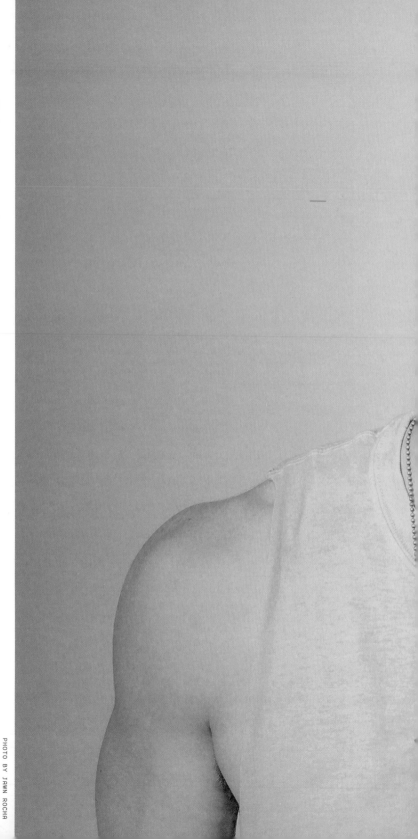

"When the hair has lifted, shampoo and then dry the hair. Apply the Manic Panic purple colors you're going for—like Electric Amethyst, Mystic Heather, Purple Haze, Ultra Violet, and so many more—and leave on for thirty minutes or so. The longer the better. Manic Panic is like a conditioner with color because it treats the hair! After you let it sit and absorb, rinse with cool water and then condition. The best trick is to add some Manic Panic purple to your shampoo, so you can wash, tone, and reapply color to your hair all at the same time!"

CHECK OUT THE ORIGINAL BLEACH BOY AWSTEN KNIGHT, LEAD SINGER OF WATERPARKS, IN A CUSTOM COLOR COLLABORATION WE CREATED TOGETHER CALLED KNIGHT BRIGHT PURPLE, AVAILABLE EXCLUSIVELY AT HOT TOPIC STORES IN OUR FORMULA 40 RANGE.

PHOTO BY JAWN ROCHA

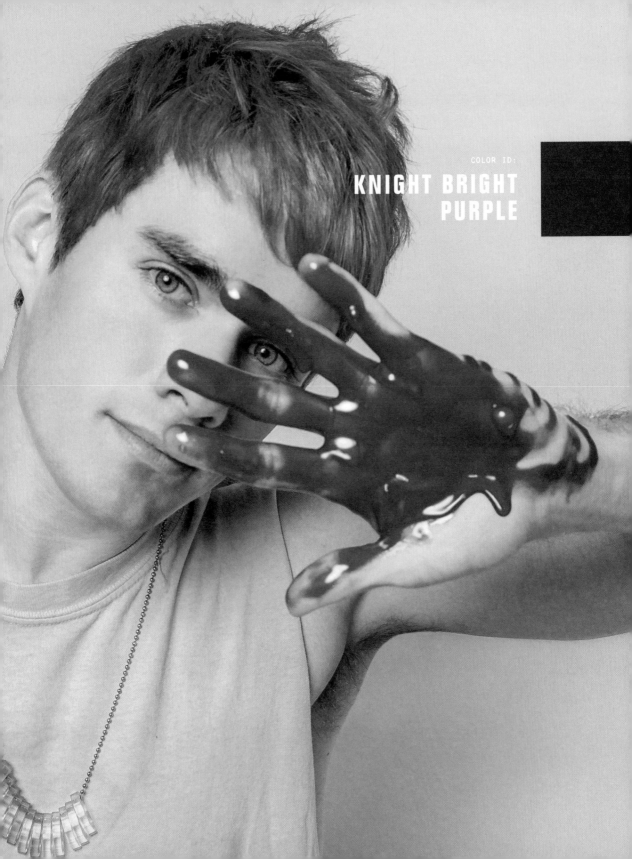

COLOR ID:

**KNIGHT BRIGHT
PURPLE**

DANIEL CORREA AND CLAUDIA HERRERA
PROVIDE THE PERFECT EXAMPLE OF WARM
VS. COOL PURPLE USING MANIC PANIC
PROFESSIONAL COLORS.

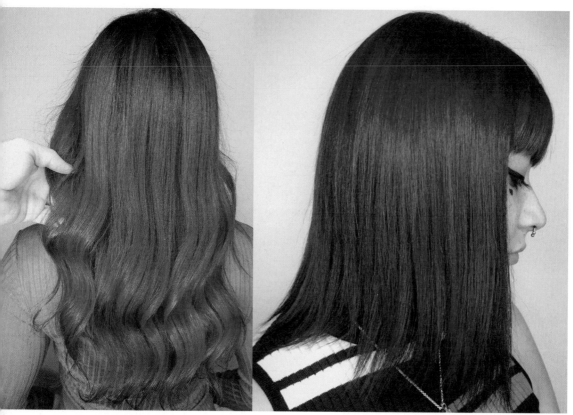

PHOTOS BY (LEFT) DANIEL CORREA
AND (RIGHT) CLAUDIA HERRERA

RED HOT CHILI PEPPERS' FLEA OVER THE YEARS HAS COLORED HIS HAIR EVERY COLOR OF THE RAINBOW. SEEN SPORTING PURPLE IN PARAGUAY, HE SAID, "ANYTHING WORTH DOING GOOD TAKES A LITTLE CHAOS."

DYEING GRAY HAIR

You'd think that natural gray or white hair would be an ideal canvas for hair color since it's naturally light, and sometimes it can be. However, gray hair can be very resistant to hair dye. It often needs to be prelightened or otherwise processed in order for vibrant colors to work best.

If you don't want to prelighten and your hair is resistant, darker colors can be used to tint gray hair. They'll eventually fade into a nice pastel. Lighter colors may add a pretty, pale hue. Please note that results may vary based on the porosity and shade of the gray hair (the whiter the hair, the more pure the tone), but we recommend using heat from a blow-dryer while processing. Always do a color test strip to avoid surprises!

Manic Panic is for everyone! You're never too young, and you're never too old!

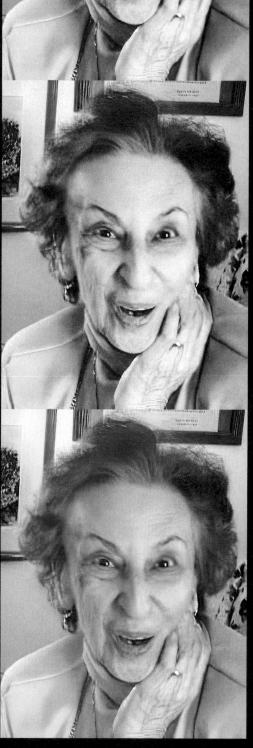

PHOTO COURTESY OF ROSE PAUL

TO COMBAT FEELING INVISIBLE LATER IN LIFE,
THE TRULY AMAZING ROSE PAUL DYED HER HAIR PURPLE,
REINVENTED HERSELF AS PURPLE ROSE, AND QUICKLY
BECAME THE CENTER OF ATTENTION.

5

HOW A SUBCULTURE BECAME A LIFESTYLE:

FROM EXTREME TO MAINSTREAM

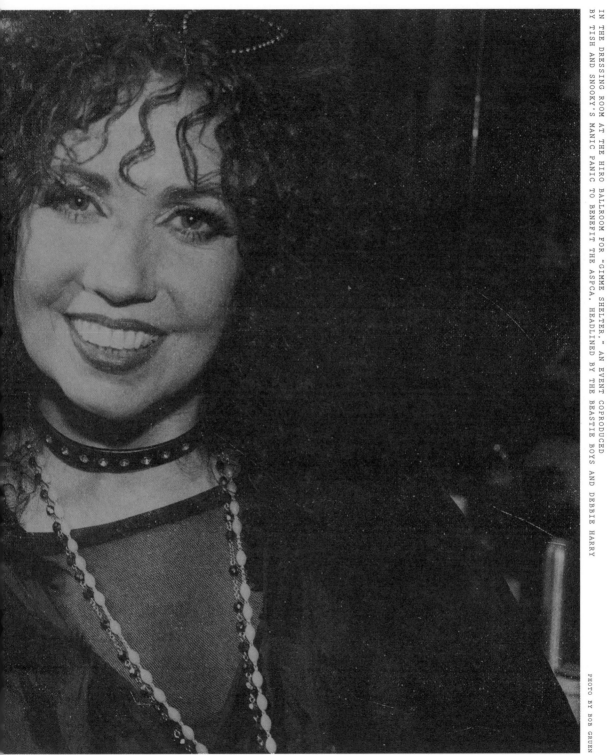

IN THE DRESSING ROOM AT THE HIRO BALLROOM FOR "GIMME SHELTER," AN EVENT COPRODUCED BY TISH AND SNOOKY'S MANIC PANIC TO BENEFIT THE ASPCA, HEADLINED BY THE BEASTIE BOYS AND DEBBIE HARRY

PHOTO BY BOB GRUEN

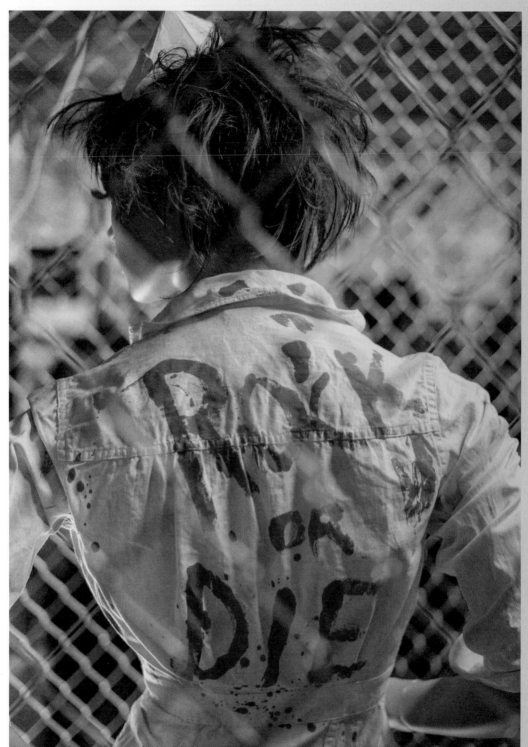

I THINK I WAS, LIKE, ELVIS PRESLEY ONE YEAR. MY SISTER DYED MY HAIR WITH MANIC PANIC. IT WAS AWESOME.... SOMEONE ASKED ME THE OTHER DAY WHY I AM AN ACTOR—THE ANSWER WAS "THAT'S BECAUSE MANIC PANIC HAD ITS WAY WITH MY BRAIN!"

—JAKE GYLLENHAAL

The new decade brought a new attitude toward hair color. Gone were the days when bold, vivid, and supersaturated hair colors were only seen on the heads of anime characters, punk rockers, or drag queens. Through the 2010s, A-listers such as Katy Perry, Rihanna, Kim Kardashian, Lady Gaga, and Cardi B have gone viral with lucid locks, but you didn't have to be a star to rock these hues.

Not surprisingly, bright hair shades made their way onto the catwalk as well, most noticeably with models Charlotte Free for Vivienne Westwood in 2011, Fernanda Ly for Louis Vuitton in 2015, and Kendall Jenner for Karl Lagerfeld in 2018. Neon mops have since been seen swinging down the runways of major houses like Jeremy Scott, the Blonds, Meadham Kirchhoff, Marc Jacobs, and Manish Arora, igniting an entirely new set of hair trends in both the fashion and beauty worlds.

This wider exposure led new generations to adopt a look once thought shocking. Millennials may be one of the most colorful and expressive generations to date, with some even building an entire social media identity and career out of their colorful hair, which garners them hundreds and thousands of followers.

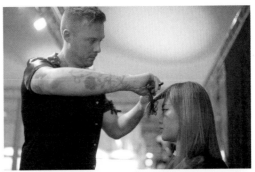

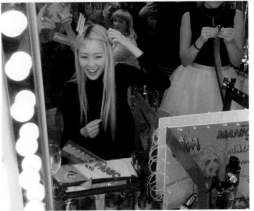

TOP
STYLIST STEVEN AUSTIN CREATED THIS MULTI-COLORED MELT USING MANIC PANIC PROFESSIONAL.

BOTTOM
IN 2015, WE DID A COLLABORATION WITH THE LIVE-ACTION REVIVAL OF JEM. AT THE LAUNCH PARTY, WE HAD FERNANDA LY FLAUNTING THE FABULOUS JEM-AMPLIFIED PINK.

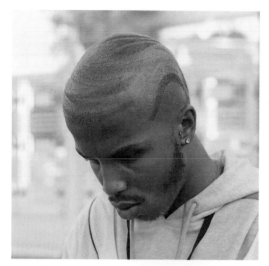

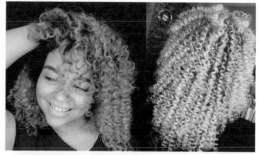

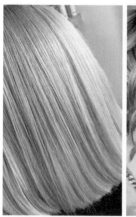

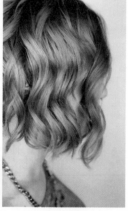

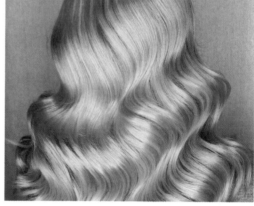

TOP LEFT
SHAROON TYLER MESMERIZES US WITH THIS INTRI-
CATE BUZZ CUT ACCENTED WITH VIBRANT SHADES OF
MANIC PANIC IN HOT HOT PINK, ATOMIC TURQUOISE,
ELECTRIC LIZARD, AND ULTRA VIOLET.
PHOTO BY SHAROON TYLER

MIDDLE FAR LEFT
JAYEL DIANE CREATED THIS AMAZING OPALESCENT
RAINBOW USING MANIC PANIC PROFESSIONAL'S
PUSSYCAT PINK, CELESTINE BLUE, AND BLUE BAYOU.
PHOTO BY JAYEL DIANE

MIDDLE NEAR LEFT
MANIC PANIC'S SARAH BRUCAS DYED HER OWN HAIR
USING ALIEN GREY CLASSIC CREAM.
PHOTO BY RENAN BARROSO FOR MANIC PANIC

BOTTOM LEFT
MANIC PANIC PRO EDUCATOR CHRISTIANA SAYYAH CREATED
A PASTEL PRISM USING BLUE BAYOU, VELVET VIOLET,
SERPENTINE GREEN, AND THE PRO PASTEL-IZER.
PHOTO BY CHRISTIANA SAYYAH

TOP RIGHT
CHRISTIANA SAYYAH AND VIKI SCISSORHANDS MADE
THESE LUSCIOUS CURLS EVEN MORE VIBRANT BY
USING MANIC PANIC PRO PASTEL-IZER TO CREATE
PASTEL AND PLATINUM STREAKS.
PHOTOS BY (LEFT) CHRISTIANA SAYYAH AND (RIGHT) VIKI SCISSORHANDS

BOTTOM RIGHT
STYLIST LAURA CHRISTOPHER WOVE STREAKS OF
PINK INTO THIS GORGEOUS LOOK USING PROFES-
SIONAL PUSSYCAT PINK + PRO PASTEL-IZER.
PHOTO BY LAURA CHRISTOPHER

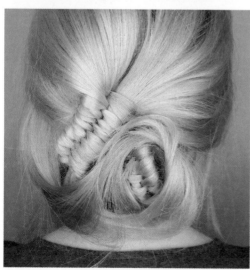

This widespread popularity has meant that wild hair colors were no longer taboo. As pioneers and authorities on the subject, Tish and Snooky, dubbed "the Queens of Creative Hair Color," became the go-to interview on the subject. As trendsetters, they were also working to perfect the formula for their brand-new products, the Manic Mixer Pastel-izer and the Creamtone Perfect Pastel formulas.

Before launching the Pastel-izer in 2015, the only way to soften Manic Panic's bright colors was to add conditioner, which caused the color to fade faster and could result in patchiness. Snooky says, "Pastel-izer was an idea that Tish had many years ago." The first of its kind, the award-winning product allowed users to get a totally customizable look, depending on how much of the colorless cream was added.

Creamtones, named after a three-piece a capella act Tish and Snooky had with their friend Diana Mae Munch in the 1990s, were Manic Panic's first foray into pastel shades.

These launches led to a surge of pale, My Little Pony-esque dos and amazing ombré effects popping up all over social media, magazine editorials, and popular beauty sites.

Manic Panic is constantly launching new and exciting colors. Tish says, "We have more colors than any other creative hair color company in the world and more possible combinations than pizzerias in Brooklyn." Snooky explains that "when we like a color, we match it up with Pantones, and then work directly with a lab to formulate it. We're very hands-on and involved when it comes to a new color because we want it to be as perfect as possible and exactly how we want it." Recent hair color trends have leaned toward the gray side of the spectrum, influencing the success of shades like Alien Grey (maybe that can go to Mars!), Amethyst Ashes, Blue Steel, and Silver Stiletto.

Not only are Manic Panic's hair colors iconic, but so are the color names: "Back in 2004, Kate Winslet starred in *Eternal Sunshine of the Spotless Mind*. Her hair was dyed using multiple shades of Manic Panic, of which her character said, 'This company makes a whole line of hair color with equally snappy names... That would be a job, coming up with those names.' And it is a job—it's our job!"

"We come up with all the names for our hair dyes ourselves, except for Amethyst Ashes, which was a contest we held for our fans to name the color," Tish explains. "Most of the time when we're naming a product, it relates to music or something we love. I personally like Vampire Red; it's my favorite." Snooky replies, "Voodoo Blue is my favorite—that, or Purple Haze is a fun name, too. Maybe one day we'll name a color Blue Coupe, in honor of the band we currently sing with alongside Dennis Dunaway [Rock and Roll Hall of Famer of the original Alice Cooper group] and Albert and Joe Bouchard of Blue Öyster Cult."

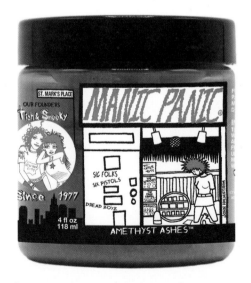

FOR OUR FORTIETH ANNIVERSARY WE RELEASED A LIMITED-EDITION COLOR THAT WAS NAMED BY OUR DYEHARDS. THEY OVERWHELMINGLY CHOSE AMETHYST ASHES, AND WHEN THE INITIAL LIMITED ORDER RAN OUT, WE MADE IT A PERMANENT FIXTURE IN OUR COLOR LINE. WE EVEN GOT ILLUSTRATOR JOHN HOLMSTROM TO DESIGN THE LABEL FOR US.

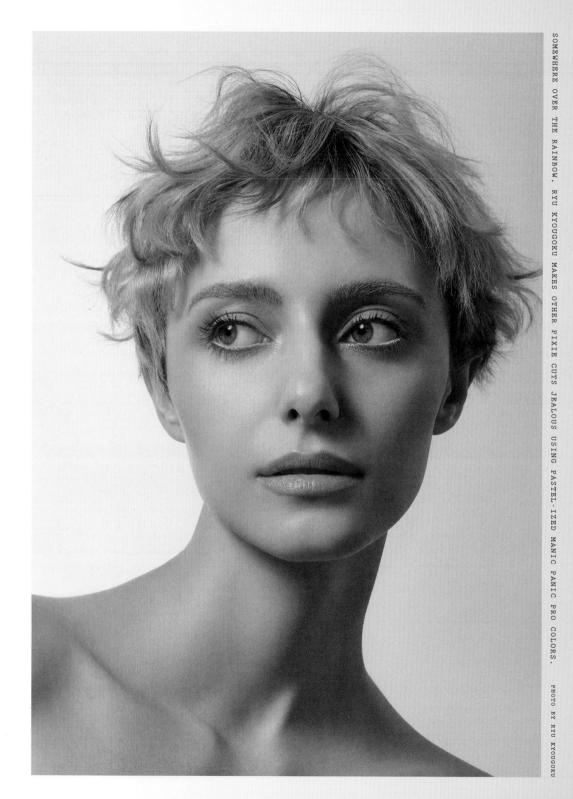

SOMEWHERE OVER THE RAINBOW, RYU KYOUGOKU MAKES OTHER PIXIE CUTS JEALOUS USING PASTEL-IZED MANIC PANIC PRO COLORS.

PHOTO BY RYU KYOUGOKU

TISH AND SNOOKY'S COLOR HISTORY

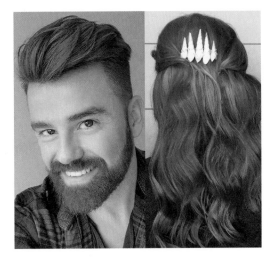

LEFT
HAIR: STEVEN AUSTIN.
PHOTO BY STEVEN AUSTIN

RIGHT
HAIR: OLIVIA FINAMORE.
PHOTO BY OLIVIA FINAMORE

For Manic Panic Dyehards, there are none more experienced than Tish and Snooky, each of whom has had her own hair color journey throughout the years.

"In the late '70s and early '80s, my hair was mostly a blend of fuchsias and reds, and once in a while purple. I just loved mixing reds and fuchsias together!" Tish exclaims. "Later on in the '90s, I went through one period when I did greens, teals, blues, and purples—a bit on the mermaidian side!

"Throughout the years I've done stripes. I'd start out by bleaching about one inch of root at my part, then I'd leave an inch of dark hair and bleach the next inch, repeating until I got to the bottom of my head, resulting in amazing horizontal stripes. My husband, Peter, has been nice enough to help with the back. After I washed out the bleach I'd then put pink or red on top and have Manic striped hair. That's one of my favorite looks—I did it back in the '70s, and then about every ten years or so I do it again. At one point I had dark green hair, light bright orange, I was rose gold before there was a name for it, and I've even been blond!

"It's funny how different hair colors make you *feel* different—when I was orange, I felt brattier; when I was blond, I felt like I could get away with more (and I did); and red hair made me feel fiery. Hair color really can change your mood and personality; it's all just color therapy. Right now I have a mix of Siren's Song, Cotton Candy Pink, Hot Hot Pink, and Fuchsia Shock in my hair, which has been my go-to blend. The only color I've ever steered away from and have not done is yellow; it just doesn't match my

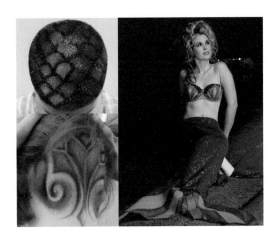

TOP LEFT
PHOTO BY SAMMY CANAVAN

BOTTOM LEFT
PHOTO BY ANGELA SKULLPTURES

RIGHT
STYLIST: THOM CAMMER.
PHOTO BY PETER PERENYI

TAKE CARE OF YOUR INNER SPIRITUAL BEAUTY. THAT WILL REFLECT IN YOUR FACE.

—DOLORES DEL RIO

personality. But hey, you never know; I might go through a yellow phase one day!"

Snooky joins in: "My gateway color was red, so I started out with the two *Bride of Frankenstein* red stripes because I loved her and thought she was so cool. Then I moved on to a full head of red and orange hair. For years and years I was some shade of red or orange; I loved fiery colors. I always wanted my hair to be the color of neon streetlights when they're just turning on at dusk. Sometimes I'd

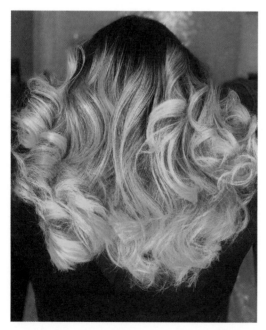

MANIC PANIC AMBASSADOR ZOE VERDEJO CREATED THIS NEON RAINBOW USING SIREN'S SONG, HOT HOT PINK, ELECTRIC BANANA, AND ELECTRIC LIZARD FOR A TRULY DAY-GLO RAINBOW. PHOTO BY ZOE VERDEJO.

bleach my roots, leave them, and then dye my hair orange to red so it would look like a sunset or a tequila sunrise—I had ombré hair before it had a name.

"When I got breast cancer in 2009, I lost all my hair after I went through chemo. Before it all fell out, we had a party and Tish cut my hair really short and we saved all my long orange-y red hair to have it sent to friends of ours in Mexico who make human hair wigs. They made me a wig out of my own hair, but I only wore it a few times because I was actually fine being bald. It's definitely a look! I realized during this time that it was only hair. My hair color may have been a reflection of me, but it didn't *define* me—it was just hair, and I really didn't care.

"When my hair grew back, I didn't feel like being fiery and having red hair anymore after the chemo, radiation, and all that heat, so I went for violet and cool shades like Ultra Violet, Purple Haze, and Electric Amethyst, and have stayed with those healing tones ever since. Occasionally, I'll add in Voodoo Blue to go back to my *Bride of Frankenstein*-inspired days, but the best part about having these hues is that our colors fade really nicely. Even if I haven't colored my hair in a long time, it still looks good because it's a pastel version!"

Tish chimes in, "People of all ages really love our hair and stop us when we're walking down the street together!"

Snooky continues: "So many people have said to us, 'We want to be just like you guys when we're your age!' We

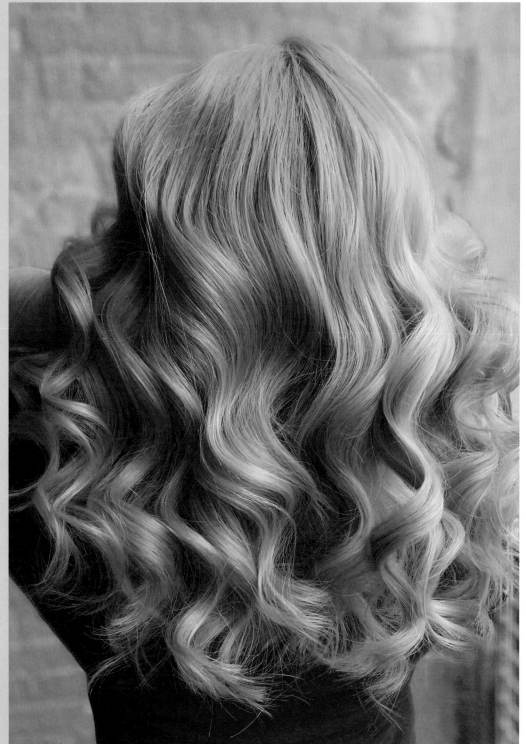

MANIC PANIC AMBASSADOR ZOE VERDEJO MAY HAVE COINED THE TERM 'GREY-NBOW' USING A MIXTURE OF SILVER STILETTO AND BLUE VELVET, WITH HOT HOT PINK MELTED INTO IT.

PHOTO BY ZOE VERDEJO

get such great feedback all the time; people always want to take pictures with us. For us, age is not a factor when it comes to dyeing your hair. Aging gracefully? That's no fun. We want to age disgracefully!"

Tish jumps in: "Yeah, we're here to embrace life. When you're older, you can get away with so much more, so you should really just go for it! When somebody young does something drastic, people get really pissed off, but when you're older, what are they going to do, yell at you?"

Snooky adds with a laugh, "And when you're older, you really don't care what other people think. Fuck 'em if they can't take a joke."

"Back in the day, unnatural hair color was more unusual to see and it really made people mad," Tish says. "Maybe they wished they could feel free enough

to express themselves but they can't, so they're frustrated! But it's also fear of the unknown, or what they don't understand. It's not just hair color. Sometimes when people see someone from a different culture, religion, skin color, etc., or someone speaking a different language and they freak out and get all weird—it's fear and just plain ol' ignorance. Why wouldn't you live and let live? That's what we do."

In the words of trailblazer Jayne County, "This is the church of rock 'n' roll, and all are welcome!" Well, this is the church of Manic Panic, and all are welcome here, too!

Snooky continues: "We used to get a lot of ridicule for how we looked, but it was just a different time period. We feel like we made it safe for everyone to have colored hair nowadays, because we took all the abuse!"

Tish and Snooky haven't just been pioneers and trailblazers in the beauty industry for more than forty years. They've been, first and foremost, creators and owners of a beauty brand that prides itself on being an ally to anyone who identifies differently. Manic Panic has always been a safe haven for the LGBTQ+ community, those who are gender nonconforming, and anyone who sees themselves as a weirdo or outcast from society. They've revolutionized the beauty industry; made a direct impact on art, music, and fashion; and weathered city gentrification trends, all while rocking creative color hair and big smiles. To know Tish and Snooky is to love them, these human rainbows, and their legacy will live in color for generations to follow.

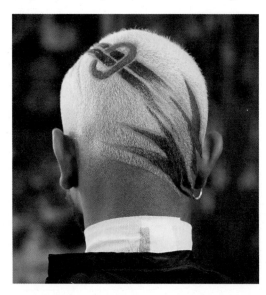

CHECK OUT THIS INTRICATE DESIGN WORK BY THE INCREDIBLY TALENTED SHAROON TYLER USING AFTER MIDNIGHT, BLUE STEEL, HOT HOT PINK, WILDFIRE, ELECTRIC BANANA, VENUS ENVY, AND PURPLE HAZE.

PHOTO BY SHAROON TYLER

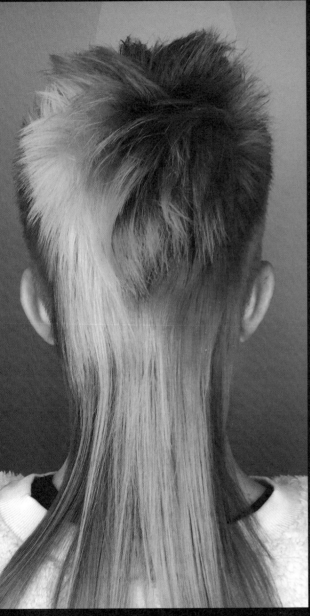

PHOTO BY KERI SCHERBRING

NOT HIDING ANYMORE

One of Tish and Snooky's favorite transformation stories comes from Dennis Preski: "I was always that 'weird' kid growing up. People would say absolutely terrible, nasty things to me... I remember having people scream 'faggot' at me before I even knew what the word meant. . . Every time I tried to stand up and be proud, and speak up for myself, someone would do something to make sure I knew how worthless I was, how lesser I was. I begged my mom for highlights for years and years, and she had finally given in, not knowing the entire time that I planned on covering that blond with Manic Panic.

"And once I finally did it . . . it was like I was untouchable. Like nobody could hurt me ever again. Oh, I'm that weird Goth kid? Yeah, I know, look at my hair. Oh, you're going to call me queer? Try again, honey, what else is new? Dyeing your hair is so much more than just changing your appearance; it changes your whole outlook on life. Everything I had been trying my best to hide, I wasn't hiding anymore and hell to anyone who was going to try and make me. I won't pretend that it was all rainbows and smiles from that point out, but from then on, it was like I had a magical barrier around me. I had taken the power away from everyone who tried to hurt me, who tried to make me feel like I didn't belong, and I had gained a brand-new power I didn't realize I could ever have—I loved myself.

"I think I might have been happier than any-one when I was asked to be an ambassador, and eventually an educator, for Manic Panic, because I want to be there for those weird little kids like me. Those punky, Gothy, queer-as-all-get-out kids who need a friend."

DOYLE WOLFGANG VON FRANKENSTEIN AND ALISSA WHITE-GLUZ.

PHOTO BY JEREMY SAFFER

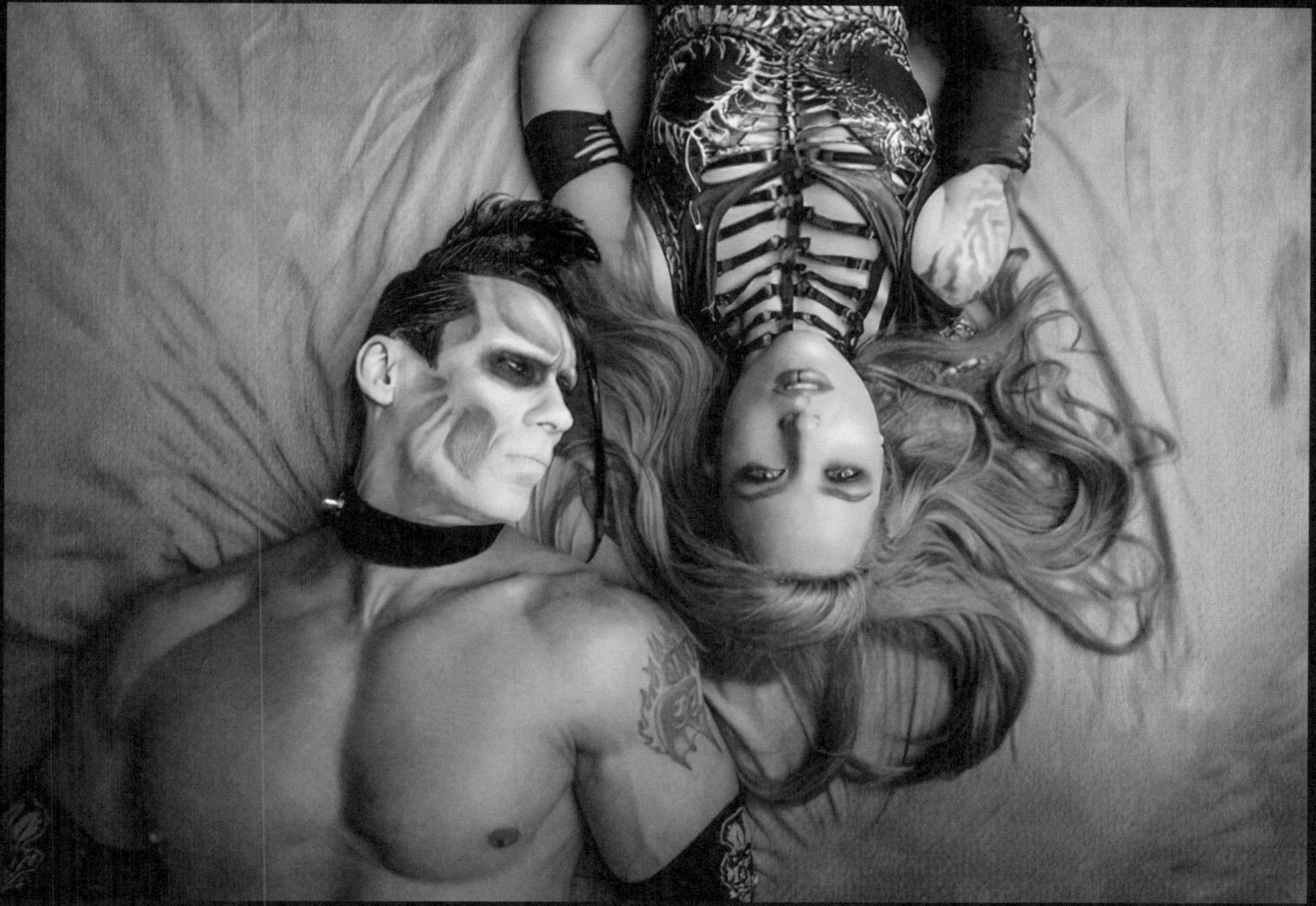

TESTED ON CELEBRITIES, NOT ANIMALS, SINCE 1977

Tish and Snooky have loved animals even longer than they have loved hair color. One of the many animals they rescued was Thumper, a cat they found behind the Manic Panic store, who was renowned for having seven toes on each foot! When they began manufacturing hair color, animal testing was still the norm. "Needless to say, we were horrified," says Tish. They were early advocates for alternative ways of testing long before it became mainstream. "We've made it our mission to improve the lives of animals everywhere by making our hair color vegan and cruelty-free since Manic Panic's inception, by donating to various animal rights and rescue organizations each year, and by rescuing animals ourselves on the street whenever and wherever we may find them."

Animal organizations are just some of the many charities that Manic Panic supports. Through their Dye for Peace® initiative, 15 percent of their profits are donated to a wide variety of charities annually.

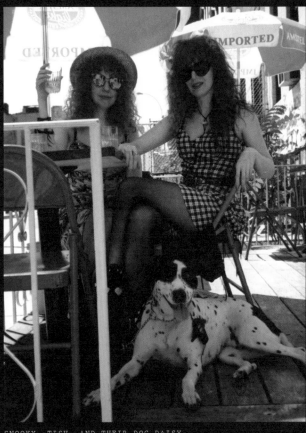

SNOOKY, TISH, AND THEIR DOG DAISY
(ONE OF THEIR MANY RESCUES!) ON
ST. MARKS PLACE IN THE EARLY '90s.

PHOTO BY PETER PERENYI

ALISSA WHITE-GLUZ,
LEAD SINGER,
ARCH ENEMY

They always say having crazy hair is a phase—
I always disagreed. Now, having spent more of
my lifetime as a Dyehard than not, I'm pretty
confident I was correct! Hair is a crowning
glory, a true vehicle of

ARTISTIC EXPRESSION.

I'm so happy that Manic Panic gave me the opportunity to decide what colors I want framing my
face without harming animals. Finding a vegan
hair dye was hard back in the 1990s when I started
my blue journey, but luckily the brightest blues
were already all cruelty-free and vegan thanks
to Manic Panic!

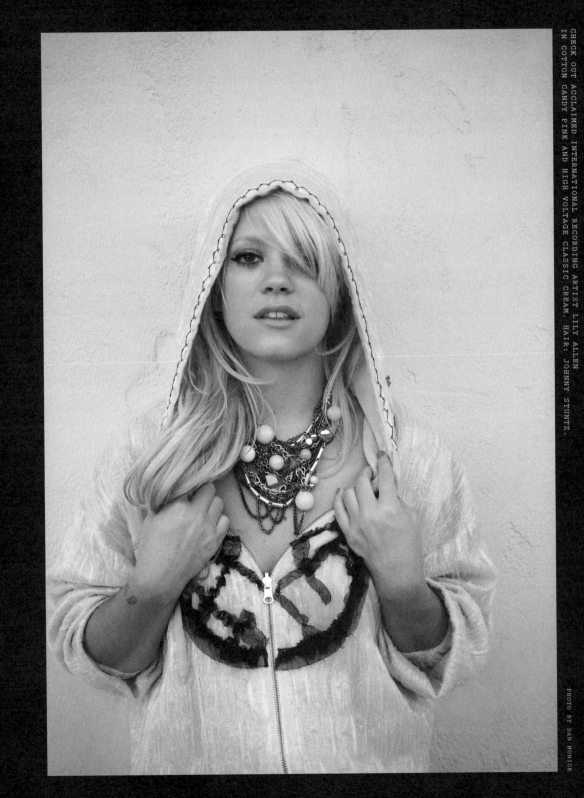

CHECK OUT ACCLAIMED INTERNATIONAL RECORDING ARTIST LILY ALLEN IN COTTON CANDY PINK AND HIGH VOLTAGE CLASSIC CREAM. HAIR: JOHNNY STUNTZ.

PHOTO BY DAN MONICK

PASTEL DREAMS, NEON NIGHTS

COLOR GUIDE

COTTON CANDY PINK	ELECTRIC BANANA	ELECTRIC LIZARD						

MANIC PANIC CREAMTONE PERFECT PASTELS

ELECTRIC TIGER LILY	HOT HOT PINK	MERMAID	AMPLIFIED CORALLINE DREAM	BLUE ANGEL	DREAM-SICLE			

MANIC PANIC GLOWS

PRETTY FLAMINGO	RED PASSION	SIREN'S SONG	FLEURS DU MAL	SEA NYMPH	VELVET VIOLET	PUSSYCAT PINK	BLUE BAYOU	RED VELVET

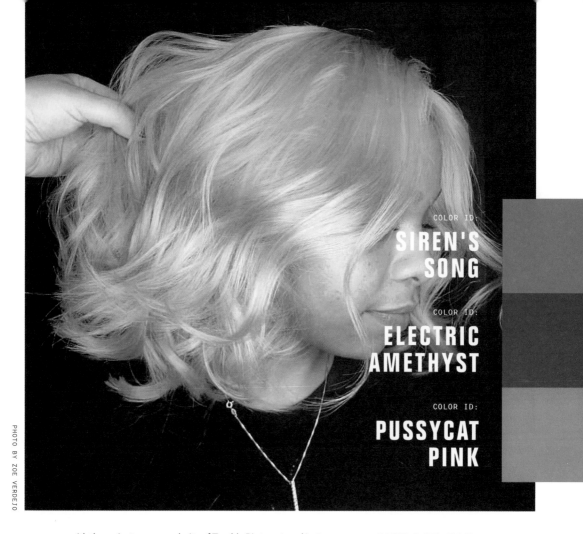

COLOR ID:

SIREN'S SONG

COLOR ID:

ELECTRIC AMETHYST

COLOR ID:

PUSSYCAT PINK

With the mainstream popularity of Tumblr, Pinterest, and Instagram, it's not uncommon to see hashtags such as #pastelgoth, #mermaidhair, or #softgrunge on photos of beautifully dyed pastel and neon hair on people all around the world. Pastel hair has been seen on everyone, including Kylie Jenner, Sky Ferreira, Elle Fanning, and Zayn Malik. On the other side of the saturation spectrum is neon hair, which has been spotted on the likes of Lady Gaga, SZA, and Nicki Minaj.

Hair colorist William Scott Blair effortlessly breaks down how to achieve both pastel and neon hair using Manic Panic's most popular shades.

"Pastel hair is tricky. Most tones of pastel, especially cooler tones, require that you lift the hair as much past yellow/orange as possible to avoid the underlying pigment making your desired result look muddy.

"For example, if you want a very light pastel blue, you have to make sure that you don't have any yellow in the hair or else it will look green. Once you've lifted the hair enough, I suggest using Virgin Snow or Silver Stiletto to tone out as much warmth as possible, and then I would use the Manic Mixer Pastel-izer with any of the colors to reach your desired result.

STYLIST ZOE VERDEJO CREATED A BEAUTIFUL STUDY IN CONTRASTING PINK AND MINT USING SIREN'S SONG + PASTEL-IZER, AND FOR THE ENDS SHE USED ELECTRIC AMETHYST + PASTEL-IZER AND A DAB OF PUSSYCAT PINK.

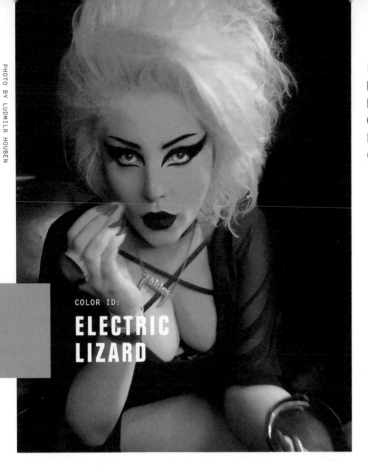

COLOR ID:

ELECTRIC LIZARD

LUDMILA HOUBEN ROCKS A RADIANT BEEHIVE WITH OUR UV-REACTIVE ELECTRIC LIZARD CLASSIC CREAM.

"Or, you can even use their Creamtones line, which come in different pastel shades—just leave it on for fifteen to thirty minutes and then rinse. Even though it doesn't seem like it, pastel hair is relatively low commitment. So for someone who is blond normally and wants a little bit of fun for a month until the color rinses out to feel different and cute, pastel hair is a perfect solution.

"I've been working with singer Melanie Martinez for about five years now. One of the true joys of my life is helping to bring her visions for herself and her hair and have it correspond to her music and the stories she tells. I loved when we did a bob and it was pastel pink with a clear line of pastel blue in the bang and at the end of the bob. Lately we've been doing barely there, muted pastel pinks, mauves, and violets. It's very much a nod to the vintage aesthetic that inspires her. One of Melanie's favorite Manic Panic shades is Pretty Flamingo; we've gone through many, many bottles of it in the past.

"When it comes to dyeing your hair neon, though, it's the same prep that's involved for going pastel. After you lighten your hair, chose from one of Manic Panic's neon shades—like Electric Banana, Electric Tiger Lily, Electric Lizard, Pretty Flamingo, or Electric Lava—and leave on the hair for about twenty minutes before rinsing. The neon hues absorb much faster on the hair, so you don't need to leave it in for as long, and the best part is that they're super longwear, so you won't have to reapply as often as the pastels."

★ HOT TIP

COLORIST CHELSEA MANFRE RECOMMENDS ALWAYS PUTTING PASTEL-IZER IN THE BOWL FIRST, THEN MIXING THE DARKER COLORS IN SLOWLY TO CREATE THE PERFECT BLEND.

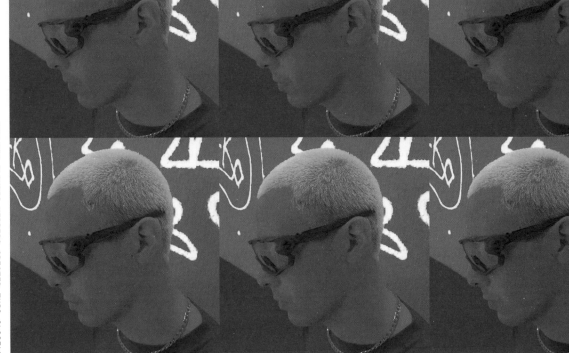

PHOTO BY CLAUDIA HERRERA

HOW TO REMOVE OR FADE COLOR FROM YOUR HAIR

If for any reason you want to remove or fade color from your hair (and we can't imagine why you'd want to, except to change to a new color!), here are a few options that can help:

- HOT-OIL HAIR TREATMENTS.

- USING ALCOHOL-BASED HAIR PRODUCTS SUCH AS HAIRSPRAY, GEL, OR MOUSSE.

- WASHING AND CLEANSING THE HAIR WITH SHAMPOOS THAT CONTAIN SULFATES, ESPECIALLY THOSE MARKED AS ANTI-DANDRUFF, CLARIFYING, OR DEEP CLEANSING.

- EXPOSURE TO WATER AND SUNLIGHT.

- CHEMICALS, LIKE CHLORINE, FOUND IN THE WATER OF A SWIMMING POOL OR HOT TUB, AS WELL AS SALT WATER FROM THE OCEAN.

- SPRINKLE A TEASPOON OF BAKING SODA INTO YOUR SHAMPOO, GENTLY KNEAD IT INTO THE HAIR, THEN RINSE IT OUT WITH WARM WATER.

RAINBOWS AND OMBRÉ: ALWAYS ON TREND

COLOR GUIDE

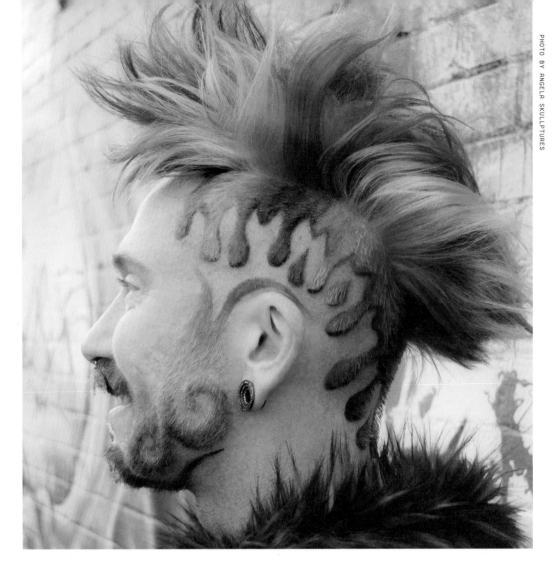

PHOTO BY ANGELA SKULLPTURES

CHECK OUT AUSTRALIAN BRAND AMBASSADOR MYKEY O'HALLORAN IN THIS UNIQUE RAINBOW-DRIP CUT AND COLOR JOB BY ANGELA SKULLPTURES USING OUR HIGH VOLTAGE CLASSIC COLORS IN HOT HOT PINK, PSYCHEDELIC SUNSET, SUNSHINE, ELECTRIC LIZARD, ATOMIC TURQUOISE, AND ULTRA VIOLET.

Where exactly did the rainbow hair trend come from, and who did it first? Was it glam rocker Roy Wood? Nina Hagen experimenting with multiple hair dye colors back in the 1970s? The Murmurs' 1994 self-titled album cover? *My Little Pony*? Clowns?

Regardless of who pioneered the look, one thing we can all agree on is that it's done best using Manic Panic. Intuitive hair colorist Roxie Darling dishes on how to build your own rainbow:

"To begin the process of achieving rainbow hair, you'll first want to start by using the Manic Panic Flash Lightning Bleach Kit with 30 or 40 volume.

"Next up, decide how many colors you want to have in your rainbow and put them out into bowls in front of you. Just remember that you'll get really incredible, vivid colors after you put them in your hair and they start to bleed together, so don't be afraid of colors overlapping onto each other during your application.

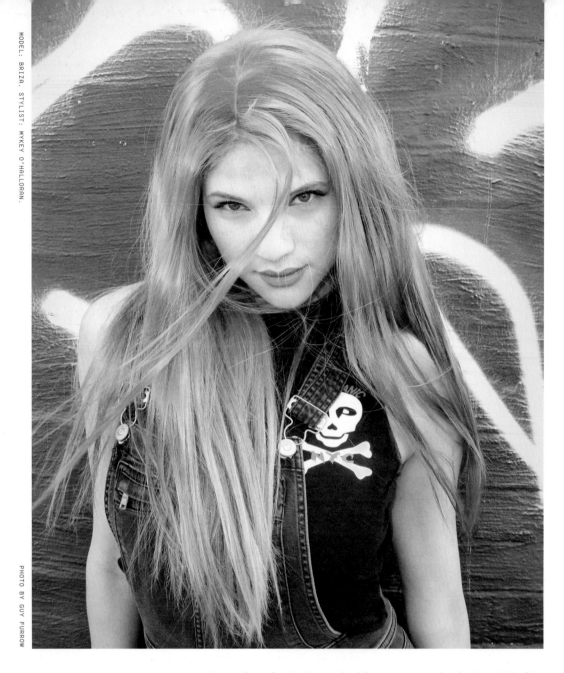

MODEL: BRIZA. STYLIST: MYKEY O'HALLORAN.

PHOTO BY GUY FURROW

MYKEY O'HALLORAN COLLABORATED WITH ANGELA SKULLPTURES ON THE ULTIMATE PRISM-PERFECT EFFECT USING THE MANIC PANIC RAINBOW DRIP KIT.

"Personally, my favorite thing to do while I'm creating rainbow hair is to think of the color wheel: I love to place opposite and complementary colors next to each other, or even on the same strand, by putting one color on the roots and then blending it out into another one throughout the mid-shaft, and then maybe even an extra color toward the ends. Or if you're looking to achieve more of a tonal rainbow—meaning all warm colors or all cool colors—the technique of putting one color on the roots and then a different color on the ends will still look really cool.

CHECK OUT THIS
INCREDIBLY
INTRICATE RAINBOW
BUZZ CUT BY STYLIST
SHAROON TYLER
USING ELECTRIC
BANANA, WILDFIRE,
ELECTRIC LIZARD,
ELECTRIC AMETHYST,
COTTON CANDY, AND
BLUE MOON.

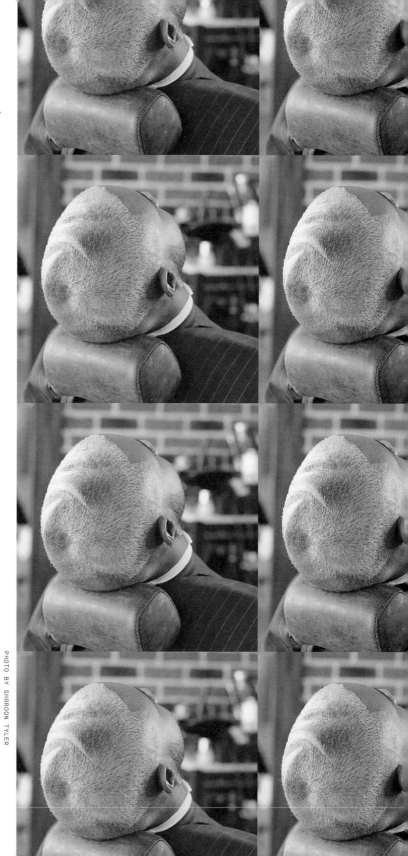

PHOTO BY SHAROON TYLER

VIKI SCISSORHANDS
PROVES YOU CAN
FIND INSPIRATION
ANYWHERE WITH
THIS GRADIENT
COLOR MELT USING
MANIC PANIC
PROFESSIONAL,
LEAVES, AND
BEETLES!

"When sectioning the hair, I also suggest making different shapes on the scalp to create the sections—for example, making a few circles on the scalp and then filling in around them—or, looking at the scalp's triangularity. My technique is to paint in all the colors in a really random, almost sporadic, but completely methodic way. Just know that rainbow hair takes a while to fully paint in.

"It's always really interesting when you leave some of the hair still blond— meaning, in between the different colors that you paint—as this allows for the light to get caught in those places and creates a really cool effect. Once you're finished painting your rainbow, let it all sit and simmer together for at least thirty minutes and then rinse with cold water, which will stop the colors from bleeding together, so it's important to follow this step!"

Another big hair trend is ombré hair. Typically, this method starts with natural root or hair color and blends into funky colors or dreamy pastels, like pink, purple, blue, and green. Dominated and popularized by celebrities like Demi Lovato, Kylie Jenner, and Rihanna, creative color ombré is the perfect alternative for anyone looking to achieve colorful locks in a more subtle, understated way. Hair colorist Tamara Kelly breaks down how one whips up an effortless ombré.

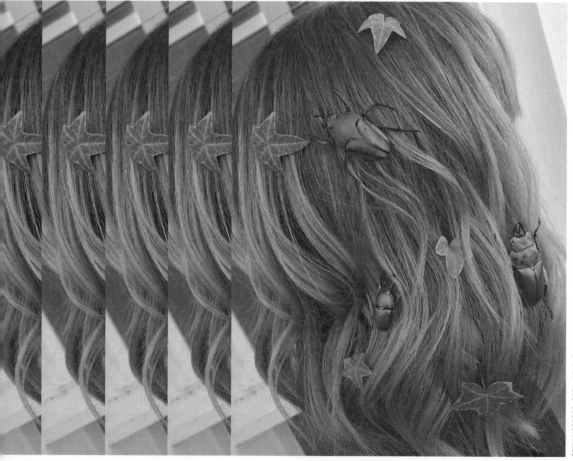

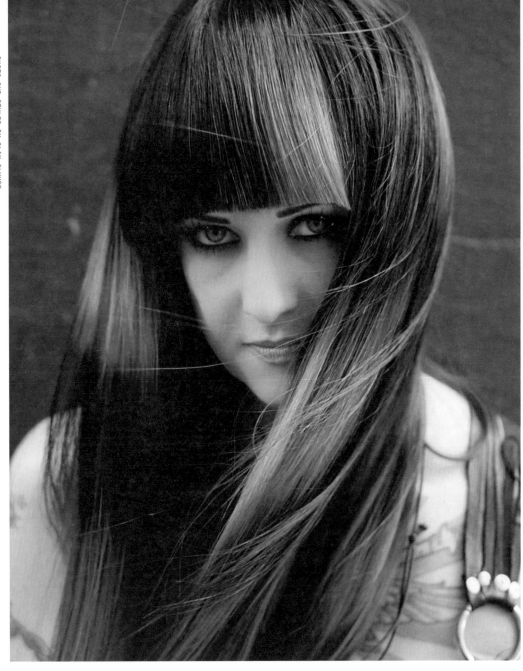

MANIC PANIC'S OWN TRINA HATFIELD WEARS A WIG INSPIRED BY FRIDA KAHLO USING MANIC PANIC PRO.

"I personally adore the ombré look, as it allows the grow out and fade of the hair color to transition into a beautiful new look. The first step to building an ombré is to start from the eyeline to jawline and map out where you'll want to start to blend so that the ombré will look intentional and not like some color service neglect. Next, I highly suggest teasing some hair through to allow a more subtle effect when applying color and blending, so it doesn't come out looking like you chopped your hair in half with a solid line in one place.

PHOTO BY RICKEY ZITO (HAIR GOD ZITO)

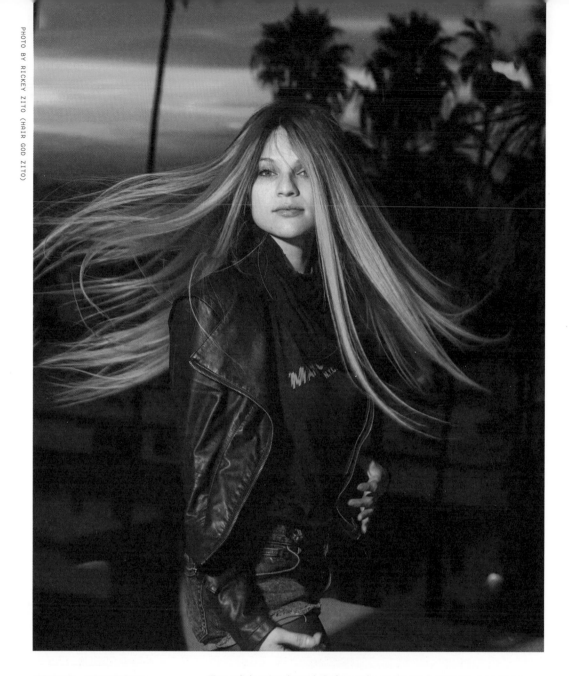

BRIZA CREATED THIS AMAZING RAINBOW WIG USING ALL MANIC PANIC PROFESSIONAL GEL HAIR COLORS.

"For prelightening the mid-shaft to ends, use the Manic Panic Flash Lightning Bleach Kit in 30 volume, checking every ten minutes, which will allow maximum lift of the color. Then you'll want to shampoo the hair, and since purple cancels out yellow, I opt for using a color-safe purple shampoo to remove any brassiness that might occur from lifting.

BRAND AMBASSADOR
STEVEN AUSTIN
CREATED THIS
MAGICAL MELT
USING OUR CLASSIC
COLORS IN CLEO
ROSE, PSYCHEDELIC
SUNSET, PRETTY
FLAMINGO, MYSTIC
HEATHER, LOVE
POWER PURPLE, AND
COTTON CANDY PINK.

PHOTO BY STEVEN AUSTIN

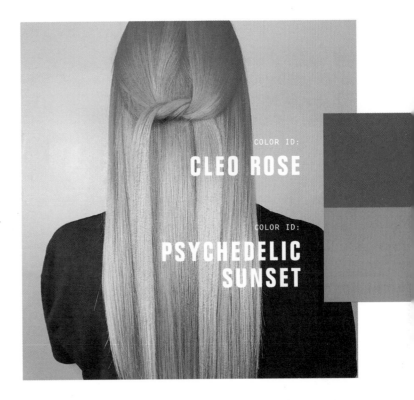

COLOR ID:
CLEO ROSE

COLOR ID:
PSYCHEDELIC
SUNSET

STYLIST GEORGIA
BELL CREATED
THIS BEAUTIFUL,
CONTRASTING
COLOR MELT USING
SUNSHINE AND
PRETTY FLAMINGO.

PHOTO BY GEORGIA BELL

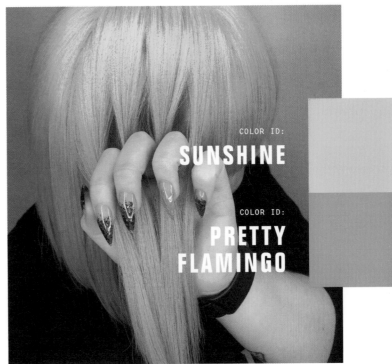

COLOR ID:
SUNSHINE

COLOR ID:
PRETTY
FLAMINGO

A CLOSE-UP ON
SOME BRIGHT CURLS
PAINTED WITH MANIC
PANIC PROFESSIONAL

PHOTO AND STYLE BY OLIVIA FINAMORE

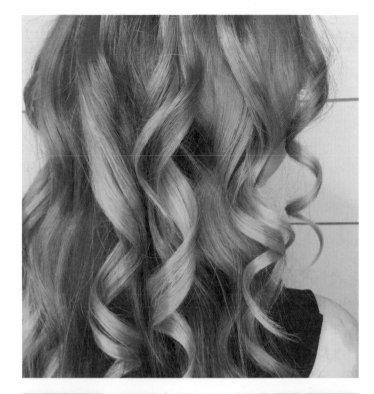

ANDRIA KAISHARIS
CREATED THIS COLOR
MELT USING MANIC
PANIC PRO COLORS
SMOKESCREEN AND
PUSSYCAT PINK.

PHOTO BY ANDRIA KAISHARIS

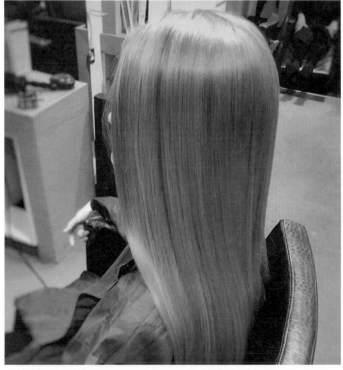

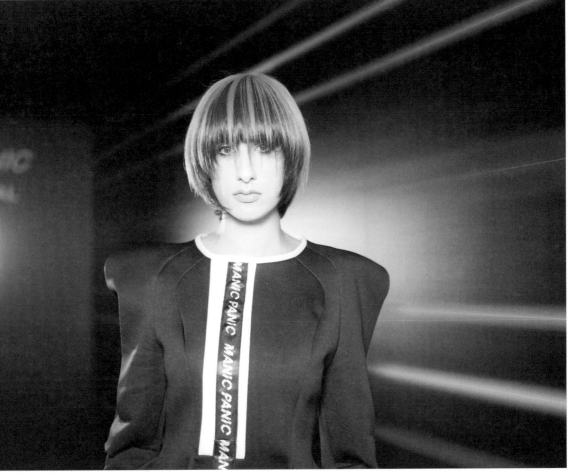

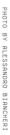
PHOTO BY ALESSANDRO BIANCHERI

MANIC PANIC EU STYLIST DEBORAH DARDI CREATED THIS INCREDIBLE CONTRASTING BOB USING MANIC PANIC PROFESSIONAL.

"If you're going for a lighter, more pastel shade toward the ends of your ombré, I recommend applying the Manic Panic Classic High Voltage hair colors on damp hair, and either getting an already pastel shade, like the Creamtones, or mixing the Pastel-izer with the color of your choice to dilute it. If you want a more intense, vivid color toward the ends of your ombré to make a great statement piece for shock and awe, I suggest applying the Manic Panic Amplified or Professional Gel Hair Color line on dry hair.

"As far as blending goes, you'll get the best results from what your eye naturally feels is the best placement, while still keeping in mind color theory. You'll apply one formula to the mid-shaft for the blend effect to be seamless, and then another formula for the end—aka the big finale! But make sure to make small subsections when applying the color formula for the most thorough application and to ensure that your saturation is perfect. Let everything sit, process, and marinate for roughly twenty to thirty minutes and then rinse out with cool water—make sure you do not shampoo. Dry and style as normal and flaunt that beautiful, blended ombré!"

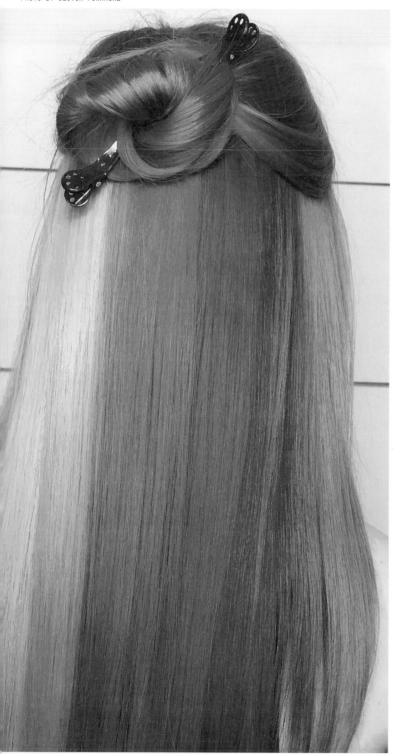

COLORIST CHELSEA
MANFRE SUGGESTS:
"ALWAYS MELT EVERY
COLOR TOGETHER
AT THE SAME TIME.
DO NOT APPLY TO
THE ROOTS AND
THROUGHOUT THE
WHOLE HEAD. GO
BACK TO APPLY THE
NEXT COLOR. THIS
ALLOWS EACH COLOR
TO PROCESS AT THE
SAME TIME FROM
TOP TO BOTTOM,
AVOIDING ANY HARSH
LINES."

LIGHT AND DARK
DUELING RAINBOWS
BY OLIVIA
FINAMORE AND MYKEY
O'HALLORAN.

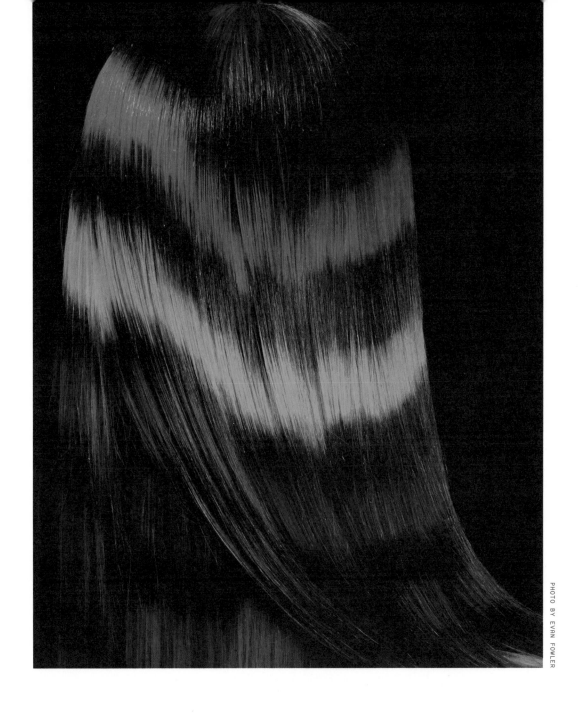

A BEAUTIFUL THING IS NEVER PERFECT.

—EGYPTIAN PROVERB

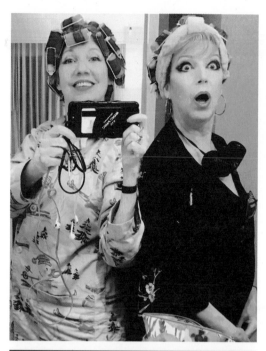

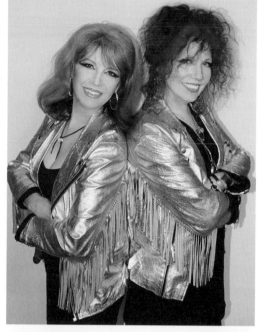

★ HOT TIP

"I DON'T COLOR INSIDE THE LINES; I COLOR MY OWN PATH. DON'T BE AFRAID TO MIX TWO COLORS TOGETHER TO GET YOUR OWN CUSTOM COLOR."

—COLORIST ANGELA BECKER

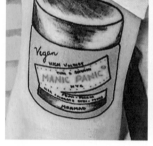

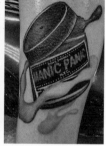

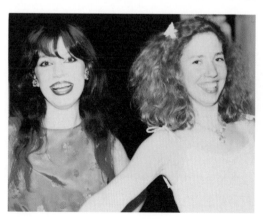

TOP LEFT
SNOOKY AND TISH AT PAJAMA PARTY IN 2018
PHOTO BY SNOOKY BELLOMO

TOP RIGHT
TISH AND SNOOKY BY MISS GUY
PHOTO BY GUY FURROW

ABOVE LEFT
MANIC PANIC TATTOO BY A FAN

ABOVE RIGHT
ANOTHER MANIC PANIC TATTOO BY ANOTHER
FABULOUS MANIC PANIC DYEHARD

BOTTOM LEFT
TISH AND SNOOKY AT CLUB 57
PHOTO BY APRIL PALMIERI

DOWNTOWN'S LAVERNE AND SHIRLEY, TISH AND SNOOKY ARE LOVABLE BOHEMIANS AND ROCK LEGENDS WHO JUST HAPPEN TO BE WORLD-CLASS BUSINESS SUPERSTARS AS WELL. THEY COLOR OUR WORLD WITH SUNSHINE WITH EVERYTHING THEY DO.

—MICHAEL MUSTO

AFTERWORD

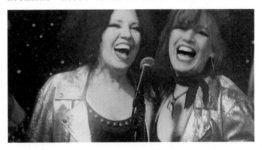

TISH AND SNOOKY IN STEVE CONTE'S "GIMME GIMME ROCKAWAY" MUSIC VIDEO BY PETER PERENYI

hat was once extreme back in the St. Marks days is now mainstream and exceeding our wildest dreams. At the dawn of shocking, vivid hair color, those brave enough to wear it would most of the time use only one color on their entire heads, or possibly try a streak or two of the same shade. Today, the planet is bursting with brightly colored coifs that are created by using a paint pallet's worth of color along with styles that have been fashioned into art statements. We had never imagined that mainstream pop icons would be rocking our colors so frequently in tabloids and websites everywhere. Nor did we expect to see mainstream celebrities work color into their hair, ranging from subtle to surreal. It has become a bona fide fashion accessory used widely and wildly. No longer is Manic Panic color limited to musicians, artists, and counterculture iconoclasts; the streets are full of people from all walks of life wearing colors that make them happy and express their inner rainbow.

So go ahead, Manic Panic your world, dare to be different, and live fast and dye your hair!

Love xoxox,

TISH & SNOOKY

CELEBRITY DYEHARDS

CELEBRITY DYEHARDS
FROM THE 2000s TO THE PRESENT DAY

- ABBEY LEE KERSHAW (MODEL)
- AMBER ROSE (MODEL)
- AMY TAN (AUTHOR)
- ANNA PAQUIN (ACTRESS)
- AWSTEN KNIGHT (MUSICIAN)
- BELLA THORNE (ACTRESS)
- BEYONCÉ (SINGER/ACTRESS)
- CARA DELEVINGNE (MODEL)
- CARDI B (SINGER)
- CAROLINE WOZNIACKI (TENNIS PLAYER)
- CHARLOTTE FREE (SUPERMODEL)
- CHLOE MACKEY (ACTRESS)
- CHLOE NØRGAARD (SUPERMODEL)
- CHRIS BENZ (FASHION DESIGNER)
- CLEO ROSE (ACTRESS)
- COCO ROCHA (SUPERMODEL)
- DANI THORNE (ARTIST/MUSICIAN)
- DASCHA POLANCO (ACTRESS)
- DEMI LOVATO (SINGER)
- DIABLO CODY (AUTHOR)
- DJ HELENA (DJ)
- DJ TIGERLILY (DJ)
- DUA LIPA (SINGER/SONGWRITER)
- ELLIE GOULDING (SINGER)
- EMILY BROWNING (ACTRESS)
- EVAN RACHEL WOOD (ACTRESS)
- FERNANDA HIN LIN LY (MODEL)
- FRANK OCEAN (SINGER/SONGWRITER)
- GEORGIA MAY JAGGER (MODEL)
- GIGI HADID (SUPERMODEL)
- GRIMES (SINGER)

- HALSEY (SINGER)
- HAYLEY WILLIAMS (SINGER)
- HEIDI KLUM (SUPERMODEL)
- HILARY DUFF (ACTRESS)
- HOLLY HAGAN (TV PERSONALITY)
- J BALVIN (SINGER)
- JAKE GYLLENHAAL (ACTOR)
- JARED LETO (ACTOR)
- JEMIMA KIRKE (ARTIST)
- JES LEPPARD (TV PERSONALITY)
- JOE JONAS (SINGER)
- JONAH HILL (ACTOR)
- JORDIN SPARKS (SINGER)
- JULIAN CASABLANCAS (SINGER)
- JUSTIN BIEBER (SINGER)
- JUSTINE SKYE (SINGER)
- KAREN ELSON (SUPERMODEL)
- KATE NASH (SINGER)
- KATY PERRY (SINGER)
- KAYA JONES (SINGER)
- KELLY OSBOURNE (SINGER)
- KELLY RIPA (ACTRESS)
- KENDALL JENNER (MODEL)
- KE$HA (SINGER)
- KIKUYO "KIKU" POLK (TV PERSONALITY)
- KIM KARDASHIAN (TV PERSONALITY)
- KREAYSHAWN (RAPPER)
- KYLIE JENNER (TV PERSONALITY)
- LADY GAGA (SINGER)
- LAUREN CONRAD (TV PERSONALITY)
- LIANA BANK$ (MUSICAL ARTIST)

- LIL DEBBIE (SINGER)
- LILY ALLEN (SINGER)
- LILY COLLINS (ACTRESS)
- LORELEI LINKLATER (ACTRESS)
- LUCY HALE (ACTRESS)
- LUPITA NYONG'O (ACTOR)
- MATTI HIXSON (TV PERSONALITY)
- MEGAN MASSACRE (TATTOO ARTIST)
- MEGHAN KING EDMONDS (ACTRESS)
- MIA (SINGER)
- MIRANDA LAMBERT (SINGER)
- NADYA TOLOKNO (ARTIST/ACTIVIST)
- NATALIE PORTMAN (ACTRESS)
- NATALIE WESTLING (SUPERMODEL)
- NEA DUNE (SUPERMODEL)
- NEON HITCH (SINGER)
- NICK JONAS (SINGER)
- NICKI MINAJ (SINGER)
- NINJA AKA RICHARD TYLER BLEVINS (INTERNET PERSONALITY)
- OH LAND (SINGER)
- OLIVIA WILDE (ACTRESS)
- RACHAEL "STEAKTOOTH" FINLEY (ACTRESS)
- RAVEN-SYMONÉ (ACTRESS)
- REBEL WILSON (ACTRESS)
- RIFF RAFF (SINGER)
- RIHANNA (SINGER)
- RITA ORA (SINGER)
- RUBY ROSE (MODEL)
- SAMANTHA NEWARK (SINGER)
- SAOIRSE RONAN (ACTRESS)
- SHARAYA J (SINGER)
- SHERYL COOPER (DANCER)
- SOO JOO PARK (MODEL)
- TALLULAH WILLIS (ACTRESS)
- VANESSA HUDGENS (ACTRESS)

- VICTORIA VAN VIOLENCE (SUPERMODEL)
- ZAYN MALIK (SINGER)
- ZOE KAZAN (ACTRESS)

CELEBRITY DYEHARDS FROM THE 1990s TO THE 2000s

- AVRIL LAVIGNE (SINGER)
- CHARLI BALTIMORE (SINGER)
- CHER (SINGER)
- CHRISTINA AGUILERA (SINGER)
- DAVEY HAVOK (SINGER)
- DENNIS RODMAN (ATHLETE)
- FLEA (SINGER)
- GREEN DAY (BAND)
- GWEN STEFANI (SINGER)
- JOSS STONE (SINGER)
- JULIETTE LEWIS (ACTRESS)
- KATE WINSLET (ACTRESS)
- KELIS (SINGER/SONGWRITER)
- MARILYN MANSON (SINGER)
- SISQÓ (SINGER)
- SYLVER LOGAN SHARP (SINGER)
- WYNONNA JUDD (SINGER)

CELEBRITY DYEHARDS FROM THE 1970s AND 1980s

- CHRISTINA APPLEGATE (ACTRESS)
- CYNDI LAUPER (SINGER)
- DEBBIE HARRY (SINGER)
- JERRY ONLY (MUSICIAN)
- KATE PIERSON (SINGER)
- MADELINE KAHN (ACTRESS)
- NORMA KAMALI (FASHION DESIGNER)
- TODD OLDHAM (FASHION DESIGNER)
- STEVEN TYLER (SINGER)

ACKNOWLEDGMENTS

irst and foremost, we want to thank our incredible mother, Estelle, for her endless and unconditional love, encouragement, selfless devotion, and total belief in us.

A special thanks to our father, Diego, for giving us our lust for life, love of singing and entertaining, and chutzpah!

Snooky: Thanks to my wonderful husband, Andy Bale, for his enduring love and support, Joe and Trudy Bale (my second set of parents), and the entire Bale family for always believing in me.

Tish: Thanks to my amazingly brilliant and talented husband, Peter Perenyi, for his love and tolerance of my busy lifestyle and for the two most wonderful guys in the world, our dear sons Orion and Peter Mac. Thanks to Gabor, Philip, and Patrick Perenyi.

We'd also like to thank:

Our grandparents Donald and Jane Mc Innes, for giving us our determination and work ethic

Our aunts, uncles and cousins:

Aunt Maddie, one of the kindest people we've ever known (who also introduced us to lipstick), Uncle Andy for his zany sense of humor, and to both of them for taking us off of our mother's hands in the summer

Cousin Jeannie for teaching us to be free spirits and to dare to be different

Aunt Harriet for lending Tish the $200 to help start the business

Uncle Ian, Aunt Sue, Cousins Ron and Alan, Uncle Walter and Aunt Ruth

Uncle Renato

Our super siblings Max, Lorena, Christian, and Romi

Gyda Gash, our forever friend and fellow rocker

Cleo Rose, our mentor and dear friend who always spoke her mind

Diana Mae Munch, our inspirational sister in song

Alan Harris for his sage advice and dedication for the past four decades

Aggie Evangelista for being our Rock of Gibraltar and always going above and beyond the beyond!

Everett Carbajal for always being the voice of reason, and protecting us from the forces of evil

Debbie Harry and Chris Stein for giving us our first big break

Gina Franklyn for her boundless energy, creativity, and sense of humor at the dawn of punk

Gorilla Rose and Tomata du Plenty for introducing us to the wacky world of off, off, off the wall Broadway!

All of our wonderful friends past and present

All our fabulous Manic-ers past and present

RuPaul for writing the foreword and helping to make the world a more accepting, fun, and fabulous place

Dinah Dunn, who came to us with her vision for this book, Lisa Tenaglia, and everyone at Black Dog & Leventhal

THANK YOU!

INDEX